# DESMOPLASTIC SMALL ROUND CELL TUMOR

# CANCER ETIOLOGY, DIAGNOSIS AND TREATMENTS

Additional books in this series can be found on Nova's website under the Series tab.

Additional E-books in this series can be found on Nova's website under the E-books tab.

# DESMOPLASTIC SMALL ROUND CELL TUMOR

NAUSHEEN YAQOOB
DALAL NEMENQANI
HATEM KHOJA
ALI KAMRAN
SYED QASIM RAZA
FUOAD AL DAYEL
ASHRAF ALI

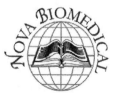

**Nova Biomedical Books**
*New York*

## NOTICE TO THE READER

The Publisher has taken reasonable care in the preparation of this book, but makes no expressed or implied warranty of any kind and assumes no responsibility for any errors or omissions. No liability is assumed for incidental or consequential damages in connection with or arising out of information contained in this book. The Publisher shall not be liable for any special, consequential, or exemplary damages resulting, in whole or in part, from the readers' use of, or reliance upon, this material. Any parts of this book based on government reports are so indicated and copyright is claimed for those parts to the extent applicable to compilations of such works.

Independent verification should be sought for any data, advice or recommendations contained in this book. In addition, no responsibility is assumed by the publisher for any injury and/or damage to persons or property arising from any methods, products, instructions, ideas or otherwise contained in this publication.

This publication is designed to provide accurate and authoritative information with regard to the subject matter covered herein. It is sold with the clear understanding that the Publisher is not engaged in rendering legal or any other professional services. If legal or any other expert assistance is required, the services of a competent person should be sought. FROM A DECLARATION OF PARTICIPANTS JOINTLY ADOPTED BY A COMMITTEE OF THE AMERICAN BAR ASSOCIATION AND A COMMITTEE OF PUBLISHERS.

Additional color graphics may be available in the e-book version of this book.

**Library of Congress Cataloging-in-Publication Data**

Desmoplastic small round cell tumor / editors, Nausheen Yaqoob ... [et al.].
  p. ; cm.
Includes bibliographical references and index.
ISBN 978-1-61470-452-2 (softcover)
1. Abdomen--Cancer. 2. Abdomen--Tumors. I. Yaqoob, Nausheen.
[DNLM: 1. Abdominal Neoplasms. 2. Desmoplastic Small Round Cell Tumor. WI 970]
RC280.A2D47 2011
  616.99'495--dc23

                                                                              2011022504

*Published by Nova Science Publishers, Inc.† New York*

# Contents

# Preface

Desmoplastic small round cell tumor (DSRCT) is a unique, highly aggressive neoplasm with characteristic topographic, histologic, immunohistochemical, cytogenetic and molecular features. It chiefly affects adolescent males and young adults and most frequently presents as a large abdominal mass with widespread peritoneal involvement at the time of diagnosis. Histologically, it is composed of nests of small, undifferentiated round or oval hyperchromatic cells embedded in abundant desmoplastic stroma. Co-expression of epithelial, mesenchymal, and neural antigens in the same cell provides evidence of origin from a primitive pluripotent stem cell with multiphenotypic differentiation. It has t(11, 22) (p13;q12) translocation, leading to a fusion of the N-terminal domain (NTD) of Ewing's sarcoma gene (EWS) to the C- terminal DNA binding domain of Wilms' tumor suppressor gene, WT1. The clinical, histologic and molecular features of DSRCT are less stereotypic and variation in the site, morphology, fusion transcript and immunohistochemistry are well documented in literature. Sometimes histologic features are nonspecific, and immunohistochemistry and cytogenetic or biomolecular techniques are required for their diagnosis. A multidisciplinary treatment including chemotherapy, aggressive debulking surgery, radiation and myeloablative chemotherapy with stem cell rescue might be the proper approach to treat this rare malignancy and may improve progression-free survival.

**Keywords:** Desmoplastic small round cell tumor, DSRCT, histogenesis, clinical features, immunohistochemistry, morphological features, cytological features, ultrastructural features, cytogenetics, radiological features, differential diagnosis, prognosis, treatment.

# Introduction

Desmoplastic small round cell tumor (DSRCT) is a primitive polyphenotypic malignant tumor with distinct clinical, histopathological and immunohistochemical features that suggest divergent differentiation and is a highly aggressive neoplasm with poor prognosis. It is the newest member of the ever growing and evolving family of small round blue cell tumors of childhood and early adulthood. It is an uncommon neoplasm that predominantly occurs in young adult men. It usually diffusely involves the serosal surfaces of the abdominal and/or pelvic peritoneum however it can present as a single mass. It has also been described in extra-peritoneal locations. Gerald & Rosai initially described it in 1989 [1], and, in the year 1991 Gerald et al [2] reported 19 cases of intra-abdominal DSRCT. However, was also recognized in 1987 by Sesterhenn et al [3] who described 17 cases of young males with undifferentiated malignant epithelial tumor arising in the serosal surfaces of pelvis and scrotum of young males. The study by Sesterhenn from Armed Forces Institute of Pathology was published in abstract form and though it antedated the description of DSRCT it did not provide detailed information of this tumor and did not include diagnostic immunohistochemical findings.

A variety of descriptive designations have been given to this tumor, including desmoplastic small cell tumor with divergent differentiation[1], intra-abdominal desmoplastic small cell tumor with divergent differentiation

[4], malignant small-cell epithelial tumor of the peritoneum co-expressing mesenchymal-type intermediate filaments [5], peritoneal desmoplastic small round cell tumor with divergent differentiation [6].

Although it has distinctive clinical, histologic, immunophenotypic and cytogenetic features, it poses a diagnostic challenge because of similar morphological appearance to other small round cell tumors that include rhabdomyosarcoma, ewings sarcoma / PNET, neuroblastoma and lymphoma. Radiographic examination shows a mesothelial like growth pattern with extensive spread along the mesothelium lined cavities. Grossly the tumor nodules are firm to hard and are of variable size and they range in shape from plaque like to spherical. Histologically, it is composed of nests of small, undifferentiated round or oval hyperchromatic cells embedded in abundant desmoplastic stroma. Immunohistochemical staining reveals a distinct polyphenotypic pattern. Trilineage co-expression of epithelial (cytokeratin, epithelial membrane antigen), mesenchymal (vimentin, desmin), and neural (neuron specific enolase) antigens in the same cell provides evidence of origin from a primitive pluripotent stem cell with multiphenotypic differentiation. A unique reciprocal translocation, t(11,22)(p13;q12) translocation, leading to a fusion of the N-terminal domain (NTD) of Ewing's sarcoma gene (EWS) to the C- terminal DNA binding domain of Wilms' tumor suppressor gene, WT1, was identified in 1992 which has become the defining feature of this tumor.

Only limited data are available on the natural history and optimal treatment of this disease [7]. Accurate estimation of the total number of patients having this disease is difficult to assess as the same patient may be reported in more than one publication.

# Chapter I

# Histogenesis

The histogenesis of DSRCT is uncertain. The consistent immunohistochemical profile, complex phenotype and its predilection for children and young adults suggest that it may arise from a primitive pluripotent stem cell with divergent differentiation. Some authors have proposed that it is derived from mesothelial or sub-mesothelial cells and termed it as "mesothelioblastoma". Its predominant spread in abdomen and pelvis and expression of epithelial and mesenchymal antigens also support a mesothelial origin.

The mesothelial origin is not only suggested by prevalence of its main location in mesothelial cell lined surfaces (peritoneal, pleural and tunica vaginalis) but also by repeated demonstration of the chromosomal translocation involving the WT1 gene which is also expressed in primitive, developing mesothelium [76]. WT1 is expressed in tissues derived from the intermediate mesoderm, primarily those undergoing transition from mesenchyme to epithelium [76, 82]. The sub-mesothelial tissues are formed from the same splanchnopleuric intraembryonic mesoderm, which also forms the kidney. The fact that the embryonal neoplasm of this organ, that is, Wilms' tumor, shares with DSRCT the capacity for multilineage differentiation along epithelial, muscle, and neural lines may be the result of this shared embryologic or cytogenetic abnormality [44].

Further support for this hypothesis comes from the finding that this tumor expresses dot-like positivity for desmin on immunohistochemical studies as do normal mesothelial cells, sub-mesothelial mesenchymal cells, and some malignant mesothelioma [9]. However, positive immunohistochemical expression for MOC-31, BER-EP4, and Leu-M1 (usually absent in malignant mesotheliomas) and the absence of cytokeratins 5/6 and thrombomodulin (usually present in malignant mesotheliomas) are against this hypothesis [8]. Other studies have also shown that DSRCT does not react to cytokeratin 5/6 and thrombomodulin but the mesothelioma does [9].

DSRCT also show no ultrastructural features of mesothelial differentiation [10, 71, 77]. Coexpression of epithelial, mesenchymal, and neural antigens in the same cell also provides evidence that DSRCT may arise from a primitive pluripotent stem cell with multiphenotypic differentiation.

Mesothelin is a glycoprotein of unknown function strongly expressed in mesothelial cells. Although there is lack of specificity of expression of mesothelin for mesothelial origin, the expression of mesothelin in DSRCT may have some significance on histogenesis [11].

Mesothelial origin is supported by Choi et al [12] who described a case of DSRCT in a 33- year-old male having pleural and pulmonary nodules along with pleural effusion. Histology of these nodules showed that they were surrounded by single layer of mesothelial cells. The neoplastic cells were positive for EMA, NSE and desmin, with the desmin positivity in para-nuclear location. The diagnosis was consistent with DSRCT. Pleural fluid showed scattered tight nests and cords of malignant cells with numerous benign mesothelial cells. Paranuclear desmin staining of many mesothelial cells was seen identical to that seen in DSRCT. They suggest that mesothelial covering of the tumor nodules suggests that the cell of origin is normally found adjacent to mesothelial cells that are the primitive submesothelial mesenchymal cells. Also the similar paranuclear staining pattern of desmin in benign mesothelial cells and in DSRCT suggests mesothelial origin. NSE positivity in this case also supports mesothelial origin as it has been found in 96% of malignant mesotheliomas [13].

The six cases of DSRCT reported by Cummings et al [56] in paratesticular location confirm the similarity of these tumors in all serous lined sites and further bolster the argument for a mesothelial origin.

Kuhnen et al [154] recently described an incidental cystic lesion in the upper left abdomen and additional smaller solid tumor nodules in a 15-year-old boy without tumor symptoms. Histopathology of the main tumorous cystic lesion showed a flattened single-cell tumor cell component in gradual transition to stratified, papillary and truly "invasive" typical desmoplastic areas of a desmoplastic small round-cell tumor (DSRCT). The author suggested that these cystic mesothelioblastic areas probably support the mesothelial origin of DSRCT.

# Chapter II

# Clinical Findings
# and Site Predilection

DSRCT has a strong male predilection with M: F ratio ranging from 2:1 to 5:1. Approximately 200 cases have been reported in the worldwide literature [14]. It is most frequently found in the serosal surface of abdomen and pelvis however it has been described in extra-abdominal locations. Fewer than 20 cases of DSRCT arising outside mesothelium- lined sites (peritoneal cavity, pleural cavity and scrotum) have been described [16].

It can affect very young children and elderly patients as late as the seventh and eighth decade. A mean age of 18.6 years is described in the literature with the range being, 5-76 years [2, 14]. Median age at diagnosis has been reported as 14, 19 and 25 years of age in different series.Only 22 cases of intra abdominal DSRCT in adult women have been reported [15]. DSRCT in females occurs at an earlier age than in males. In the study conducted by Gerald et al, mean age of diagnosis for female patients was 4 years younger than for males [76]. It has also been described in postmenopausal women [17, 18, 19].

The tumor has the tendency to spread along the mesothelium lined surfaces. Typically it presents with widespread paraserosal masses particularly in the abdomen, pelvis, retroperitoneum, omentum and mesentry. The most common site is pelvis (62%) followed by spreading widely on the peritoneal surface (42%) [20].The abdominal mass tends to be large at presentation, upto 40 cm in some cases [14]. Most patients have disseminated widespread disease at the time of clinical presentation and the organ of origin is mostly difficult to ascertain.

Signs and symptoms are usually related to the site of involvement. Common clinical presentations are pain, abdominal distension, abdominal bloating, and palpable abdominal, pelvic and scrotal mass. Hepatomegaly is present at times with associated ascites with or without weight loss. Takahira et al [21] have reported abdominal pain in 52.1% of the patients followed by increased abdominal girth in (8.4%) and abdominal mass in 5.6%. One case has been reported in a patient with Peutz-Jeghers syndrome [22]. Lae et al [80] has described four patients presenting with umbilical hernia. Pressure effects on nearby structures may cause erectile dysfunction, intestinal obstruction, urinary dysfunction and hydronephrosis. Of the 19 patients described by Gerald et al [2], 13 had difficulty in voiding. Furman et al [23] reviewed 109 reported cases of DSRCT with few cases involving urogenital organs. The sites of urogenital involvement were pelvis, 12 patients; paratesticular region, 11 patients; Bladder, 5 patients; ureters, 3 patients; and prostate gland, 3 patients. The most frequent complaint was pain followed by mass and then signs of urinary obstruction. Murosaki et al [24] have described a case of retrovesical DSRCT with urinary frequency, peri-anal pain and anal bleeding in a 21-year-old Japanese male. This suggests that DSRCT should be included in the differential diagnosis of intra-abdominal mass with urologic symptoms.

GI bleeding was first reported in the literature by Chang et al [25] in a 27-year-old man, which was associated with tumor masses involving small and large intestines and gastric antrum directly invading to the gastric mucosa.

Cases with pulmonary and pleural involvement present with pleural effusion and chest pain.

Widespread peritoneal and omental spread can be seen with lymph node involvement and hematogenous metastases particularly to liver, lung, bone marrow and lymph nodes. The signs and symptoms are overall non-specific and non-diagnostic. DSRCT should be considered in the differential diagnosis when a young adult male presents with such nonspecific findings and radiologic evidence of disseminated disease process.

The first manifestations of a tumor primarily affecting soft tissues of the scalp were headache and weight loss, and chronic sinusitis was the first sign of an ethmoidal sinus tumor [30].

DSRCT appears to show less topographic restriction. Cases involving central nervous system [26,27,28,76], parotid [29], sinonasal region [30], sub-maxillary region [31], sub-mandibular region [97], kidney [32,33,34,35, 36,155], bone [39,40,41,42,76], extremities, lung [43,45], and pleura [12,44, 46,47,76], pancreas [48,49], lymph nodes [50], para-testicular region [2,23,52,53,54,55,56], ovary [59,60,61,62,63,64,65,156], liver, spleen, intestines, have been reported. Its rare occurrence in locations distant from the mesothelium has particularly been reported in brain, parotid, sub-maxillary location, bone and sinonasal region. Tumors present in extra abdominal location are usually less extensive although a case of sinonasal DSRCT with orbital and intracranial extension has been reported by Finke et al.

Four fully documented cases of DSRCT of the central nervous system are described in literature. Neder et al [27] have recently described two cases in a 37 and 39-year-old males respectively, arising in the cerebellopontine angle and underwent spinal dissemination.

DSRCT has been reported in kidney [32, 33, 34, 35, 36, 155]. First case of renal DSRCT was reported by Su et al [32] in a 41-year-old adult male. Tumor was discovered incidently during health examination. A notable aspect of this tumor was the presence of two aberrant EWS-WT1 fusion transcripts. The four cases of DSRCT reported by Wang et al [33] in children (Age range between 6-8 years) lacked the characteristic desmoplasia. The biologic basis for desmoplastic features of DSRCT is poorly understood. The chimeric product acts as a novel aberrant transcription factor, modulating the expression of genes that overlap with those generally regulated by WT1. Platelet derived growth factor alpha (PDGF-A) is one of the targets and is a potent fibroblast growth factor that may contribute to the development of desmoplastic stroma [37,38] An upregulated expression of PDGF-A induced by EWS-WT1 chimeric protein has been proposed to account for the desmoplastic reaction, therefore a direct correlation between the level of

PDGF-A expression and the degree of desmoplasia would be expected [37]. However, an inverse correlation between the two was demonstrated by immunohistochemistry in DSRCT and was speculated upon the existence of a complex and indirect effect of PDGF-A on desmoplasia [38]. Wang et al [33] in his study suggested a direct correlation between the expression of PDGF-A and TGF-3 with desmoplasia.

Murphy et al [39] reported first case of primary DSRCT of bone confined to right ilium with no associated soft tissue mass. The tumor involved the right iliac bone wing and the posterior aspect of the roof of the acetabulum with relative sparing of the anterosuperior part of the iliac bone and sacroiliac joint and with minimal (<5% of tumor bulk) extension into adjacent soft tissue. The previously reported case by Adsay et al [40] involved the metacarpal bones of hand involving the soft tissue of hand with secondary bone extension. Biswas et al [41] have reported DSRCT in upper and lower extremities in 2.5 and 1.5 year old females respectively. Yoshida et al [42] have also described primary DSRCT of femur in a 10-year old female with pulmonary metastases.

Parkash et al [44] have described three cases of DSRCT, primarily in the pleura. Since most of the previously reported cases involved the peritoneum or tunica vaginalis, hence, occurrence of these tumors in the pleura suggests a histogenetic relationship to the mesothelium. Patients with DSRCT of the pleura usually present with clinical, radiologic, and gross features similar to those of a mesothelioma. As a matter of fact, it has been suggested that some childhood mesotheliomas reported in the literature might actually have been DSRCT [10].

DSRCT has been reported in pancreas [48, 49]. One case of pancreatic DSRCT is recently reported with breast metastases [49]. Lymph node metastases can rarely occur in DSRCT and may represent first manifestation of the disease [50]. Metastasis to liver, bone marrow and lymph nodes has been documented in 33% of cases [51].

DSRCT is reported in the paratesticular area [52, 53, 54, 55, 56 ]. Literature review by Roganovich et al [52] has found 13 cases of primary scrotal involvement. Involvement of tunica vaginalis is also reported [56]. Most patients consulted due to the presence of testicular pain or a scrotal mass which was confirmed by ultrasonographic findings. Diagnosis of theses masses depend on histopathological evaluation. Therapeutic approaches differ however most authors agree that resection and post operative chemotherapy and radiation are the best therapeutic options. The ideal therapeutic approach for paratesticular DSRCT is debatable and different therapeutic regimens have been employed and there is no standard protocol for these patients. Most authors agree on resection and post operative chemoradiation therapy as the best therapeutic options. Paratesticular tumors can usually be completely resected however some authors recommend orchiectomy [136]. Gonzalez et al [53] have described a case of paratesticular DSRCT in a 23-year-old male located in the tail of right epididymis treated by complete resection of the mass as it was connected to the testicle through a narrow pedicle and there were no satellite lesions. It was followed by chemoradiation therapy. The patient remained free of disease in the 6-year follow-up period. Recent reviews on desmoplastic small round cell tumor affecting the paratesticular region have shown a better prognosis for these tumors at this site compared to those seen in abdomen as they become clinically apparent at an earlier stage [54]. According to the published literature, the para-testicular DSRCT behaved in a clinically aggressive fashion, in some cases producing lymph node metastases to the retroperitoneum and other sites, as well as lung metastases. However according to Roganovich et al [52] the prognosis of patients with paratesticular DSRCT may still be better. In fact out of 10 published cases of paratesticular DSRCT, 4 were alive with no evidence of disease 2.5-3 years after diagnosis at the time of being reported [52].Cummings et a [56]l presented the largest series of six cases of paratesticular DSRCT. The age range was from 17 to 37 years (Mean 28 years). Five patients presented with scrotal mass and one patient presented with testicular pain. Four tumors metastasized to lymph nodes and one patient had pulmonary metastases. In three cases numerous small nodules studded the tunica albuginea away from the main mass and in four cases the tumors extensively involved the epididymis. The testes themselves were unremarkable.

Gynecologic presentations of DSRCT are diversified. In women, DSRCT has been reported in ovary, fallopian tube, liver, lymph nodes, colon, and, very rarely, in the uterus and vagina. Church et al [57] presented a case of obstructed labor due to abdominopelvic widespread disease and multiple cystic metastases in the liver. Khalbuss et al [58] has reported DSRCT presenting as cervico vaginal mass with multiple liver metastases and raised CA 125 level of 244 IU/mL. Vaginal bleeding may be the initial presentation of intra-abdominal DSRCT with involvement of the vagina and the cervix. Bland et al [15] presented a case of 33-year-old African- American woman who presented with large omental tumor and nodules on bowel surface and tumor plaque coating the abdominal and pelvic peritoneum & uterus, six month after an uncomplicated vaginal delivery.

DSRCT may mimic an ovarian primary tumor. Hence, it should be added to the differential diagnosis of unusual gynecologic malignancies in elderly as well as younger females. Ovarian involvement by DSRCT is rare with only 10 reported cases in the literature [59,60,61,62,63,64,65,56], 3 of them have been reported in a single study. DSRCT involving ovaries is seen in young women, with age ranging from 11-27 years and the clinical presentation is non-specific. According to a study of 17 cases of DSRCT in young women, conducted by Zaludek et al [61] ovarian involvement was observed in 30% of his cases. One of the patients presented with symptoms of acute appendicitis [59]. Widespread peritoneal disease with multi organ involvement was the common clinical finding with lymph node metastases. Unilateral ovarian involvement was more frequent as seen in 7 out of 10 reported cases however DSRCT can involve ovaries bilaterally.

Another case is reported by Slomovitz et al [62] who reported ovarian involvement by DSRCT in a young female. We have also seen a case of DSRCT in a 23-year-old female [64] with bilateral ovarian masses and widespread peritoneal involvement. The patient also had raised CA-125 levels. Similar case of DSRCT with raised CA-125 levels with ovarian, omental and hepatic involvement in a young female was reported by Parker et al [65]. Reich et al [19] have described a DSRCT in a post menopausal presentation, an unusual age of presentation, mimicking a metastatic ovarian neoplasm. DSRCT may mimic an ovarian primary tumor hence it should be added to the differential diagnosis of unusual gynecologic malignancies in elderly as well as in young females.

# Chapter III

# Tumor Markers

No specific tumor markers have been described in literature for DSRCT however raised CA 125 levels have been identified in many cases. CA 125 is a high molecular weight glycoprotein and it is often present in the non-mucinous surface carcinomas of the ovary and in the adenocarcinomas of cervix and endometrium. Elevated values are sometimes found in various benign gynecological diseases such as ovarian cysts, ovarian metaplasia, endometriosis and cervicitis. It is also seen in the mesothelial cells, epithelial cells from the pancreatic ducts, bronchial tree, colon, gall bladder, stomach, kidney and breast. Although the highest values occur in patients with ovarian carcinoma, clearly elevated levels have also been shown in pancreatic, breast, colon, endometrium, fallopian tube and lung malignancies. Serum CA 125 levels have extensively been used as diagnostic indicators and therapeutic monitors in various gynecological malignancies.

Patients presenting with elevated serum levels of CA 125 antigen may potentially be misdiagnosed to have some other abdominal malignancy. An elevated serum CA 125 concentration is found in 86% patients of intra abdominal DSRCT with a median value of 200 U/ml (range 22-735) [66].This high serum concentration is attributable to the tumor cells or to the mesothelial expression of this antigen is debatable. It was proposed that the raised CA 125 levels may be related to ascites and not directly to the tumor itself [124]. Church et al [57] described a case of pelvic DSRCT in a 29-year-old woman. Serum CA 125 at presentation was 196 Kiu/l, which dropped to 6 Kiu/l after receiving chemotherapy.

Yang et al [67] reported CA 125 concentration of 882.1 U/mL (normal, <35 U/mL) in a 29-year-old patient having intra abdominal DSRCT between rectum and urinary bladder with liver and lung metastases. The serum concentration normalized to 20.7 U/ml after chemotherapy, re-elevation of the concentration was noted when the tumor grew again, thus CA 125 concentration can be used to monitor the treatment progress.

Ordonez et al [68] described the case of a 34-year-old female with DSRCT and high serum CA125 levels, which decreased after chemotherapy and surgical debulking of the tumor but rose again with recurrence of the disease process. The reduction of the patients CA 125 serum level after receiving chemotherapy and surgical removal indicates that the primary source of the antigen was in the tumor cells. He suggested that CA 125 could be used as a marker of persistent and recurrent disease in those uncommon cases of DSRCT in which there are elevated serum levels of this marker at the onset of treatment.

On the contrary, according to some authors CA 125 should not be considered as a highly sensitive marker for recurrent DSRCT. DSRCT with raised CA125 levels with ovarian, omental and hepatic involvement in a young female was reported by Parker et al [65] In this case the patient presented with elevated CA125 level of 140 U/mL, which decreased to 15 U/ml after one cycle of chemotherapy. The last CA 125 level was 11.8U/mL at which time she was discovered to have extensive peritoneal and lymph node involvement by the tumor.

Association of raised CA 125 has been reported in two cases of DSRCT in pediatric patient [62, 69] and 2 adult cases of DSRCT [68, 70]. Khalbuss et al [58] reported fifth case of DSRCT presenting as cervicovaginal mass with raised CA 125 level of 244 IU/ml.

# Chapter IV

# Morphological Features

Grossly the tumors are usually large (up to 40 cm in some cases) and are often accompanied by multiple peritoneal implants. Outer surface of the tumor is bosselated and cut surface shows gray-tan appearance with areas of necrosis and sometimes with myxoid changes.

Histologically, sharply demarcated angulated nesting growth pattern is seen, with uniform small, undifferentiated round or oval hyperchromatic closely packed malignant cells distributed in a background of desmoplastic stroma. (Figure 1) The shape of tumor cell clusters varies from round to elongate. (Figure 2) The histological appearance varies from densely cellular areas to occasional clusters of tumor cells scattered in abundant desmoplastic stroma.

The stroma is primarily fibroblastic and is largely made up of fibroblasts and myofibroblasts embedded in a matrix of loose or myxoid extracellular material (Figure 3) with variable collagen deposition (Figure 4) and a distinctive vascular hyperplasia sometimes exhibiting a lobular configuration. The tufts of blood vessels have plump endothelial and perithelial cells [2]. It is unclear that the striking desmoplasia is the result of an intrinsic property of tumor cells or just a reflection of the well known tendency for reactive proliferation of the sub-mesothelial mesenchyme.

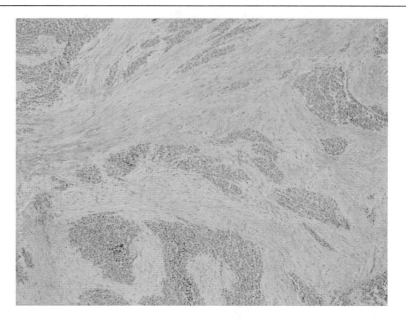

Figure 1: Sharply demarcated nests of tumor cells embedded in hypocellular desmoplastic stroma. (Original magnification 100x).

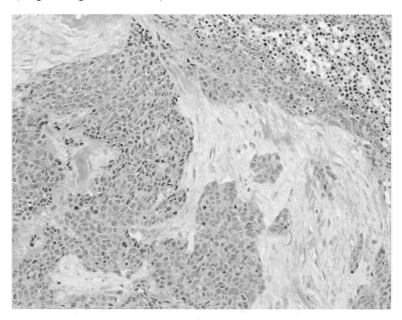

Figure 2: Note angulated nests and cords of tumor. (Original magnification 200x).

Since the distant metastases also showed desmoplasia hence the former hypothesis is favored. The striking vascular proliferation might be secondary to the secretion of angiogenic factors by the tumor cells [2]. Geographic necrosis especially at the center of tumor cell clusters (Figures 5 & 6) and cystic degeneration are common features. Necrosis is seen sometimes associated with calcific concretions [2]. Mitotic index is usually high. There is marked uniformity among tumor cells within the cluster. Nuclei are densely hyperchromatic and small to medium sized with inconspicuous nucleoli. (Figures 7 and 8) Cytoplasm is usually scanty with indistinct cell boundaries.

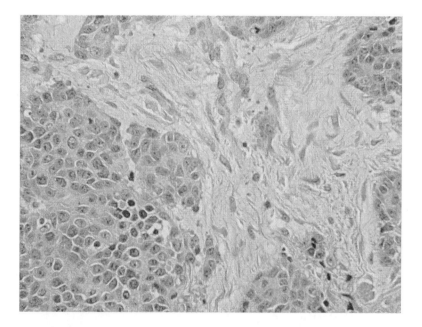

Figure 3: Fibroblastic stroma exhibiting myxoid changes. (Original magnification 200x).

The histologic variability in DSRCT is greater than believed and poses formidable diagnostic challenge. Morphological variation is well documented and is reported in upto one third of the cases [71] including tumors with no desmoplasia [33,80]. Several other atypical patterns have been described with glandular, basaloid, solid areas with very little desmoplastic stroma, pseudo-rosettes [56, 71], and even fusiform and papillary areas [73].

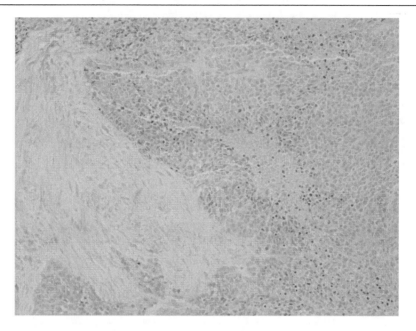

Figure 4: Variable collagen deposition is seen in desmoplastic stroma. (Original magnification x 200).

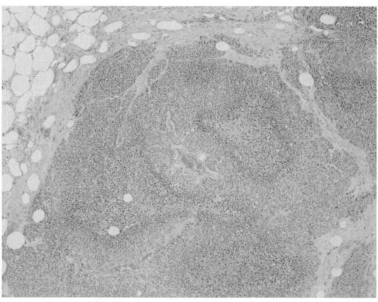

Figure 5: Areas of geographical necrosis seen at the center of tumor cell clusters. (Original magnification 200x).

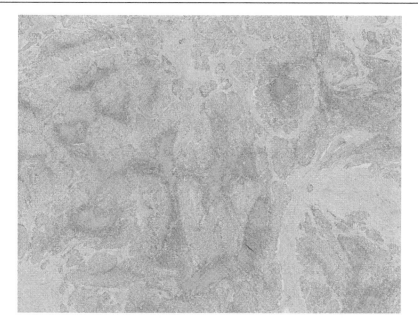

Figure 6: Areas of geographical necrosis seen at the center of tumor cell clusters. (Original magnification 100x).

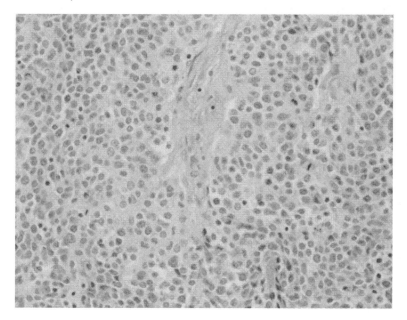

Figure 7 and Figure 8. (Continued).

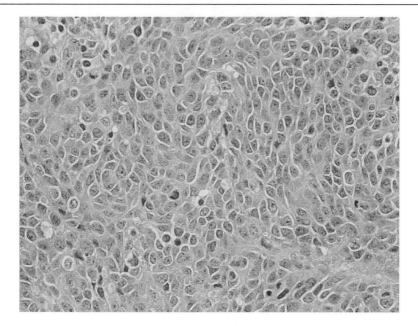

Figure 7 & Figure 8: Higher magnification showing uniform tumor cells with densely hyperchromatic nuclei and inconspicuous nucleoli and high mitotic index. (Original magnification 200 & 400x).

Various architectural patterns including rosette like structures mimicking neuro-blastoma, insula, short cords [56], tubules [56,71,74], ribbons, carcinoid like morphology, solid foci resembling transitional cell carcinoma, adenoid cystic like configuration, multicystic and anastomosing trabeculae are described. Cell morphology includes rhabdoid cells [2, 49], clear cells [2], signet ring cells [68], extensive areas of spindle cell morphology [75], squamous differentiation [49,56], and pleomorphic [2,16], bizarre large tumor cells [72]. Young et al [60] reported ovarian involvement by DSRCT and described nests of tumor clusters with peripheral palisading of basaloid cells. Alcian- blue positive myxoid matrix and PAS positive diastase resistant intra and extracellular hyaline globules were described in renal DSRCT [33]. Psammoma bodies are also described [56].

Dorsey et al [73] reported DSRCT in a 29-year-old male with a well developed epithelioid papillary growth pattern with no necrosis and mild desmoplasia. The desmoplastic stroma was pauci-cellular, limited in amount and present in areas separate from the papillary structures. Areas of back to back single cell infiltration that mimicked loblular carcinoma of breast were also seen. This different histological pattern is suggestive of morphological variation of DSRCT.

Tumors that lack classic histological features pose diagnostic challenge and definitive diagnosis depends on demonstrating epithelial, mesenchymal and neural markers and the tumor specific EWS-WT1 fusion. Zhang et al [74] reported a case of DSRCT in a 17-year-old female patient that not only had a peculiar morphology but also lacked expression of epithelial markers. It had architectural patterns ranging from microcystic areas, pseudo acini formation, trabeculae & cords anastomosing in a plexiform or filigree pattern embedded in a myxoid stroma with prominent glomeruloid endothelial proliferation and occasional thick desmoplastic septa. Mitoses were infrequent. The tumor was negative for epithelial markers however showed variable positivity for vimentin, desmin, smooth muscle actin, Neuron Specific enolase (NSE), Bcl-2, WT-1 and synaptophysin. Definitive diagnosis was made by the demonstration of characteristic EWS-WT1 gene fusion by fluorescence in situ hybridization.

Ordonez et al [68] reported a case of DSRCT with combination of several histological patterns. It showed prominent signet ring morphology which on electron microscopic studies was attributed to the coalescence of intra-cytoplasmic vacuoles combined with a progressive dilatation of the inter-cellular space resulting in displacement of the nucleus toward the periphery of cell. Signet ring cells are usually seen in various tumors due to accumulation of mucin, and, in non-mucinous tumors like lymphoma, melanoma, adenocarcinoma prostate and thryroid tumors due to large intracytoplasmic lumen, expansion of rough endoplasmic reticulum with immunoglobulin, presence of giant multivesicular body, or large lipid droplet.

The possibility that spindle cell features can be detected in DSRCT has already been reported by Lae et al [80].DSRCT with leiomyosarcoma like morphology is reported by Alaggio et al [75] who described two tumors in pediatric age group exhibiting spindle cells arranged in sheets and fascicles without desmoplastic stroma with the EWS-WT-1 7/8 transcript associated with favorable prognosis. Tumor cells were positive for cytokeratins, smooth muscle actin, desmin and muscle specific actin however were negative for

EMA. RT-PCR analysis showed EWS-WT1 fusion transcript. The EWS-WT1 chimeric protein functions as a transcriptional activator of the interleukin 2/15 (IL2/15) receptor β chain in tumor cells, whereas the desmoplastic stroma expresses IL2 and IL15, thus providing the paracrine signal for tumor cell proliferation [126].These patients are alive at 3 and 13 years after the initial diagnosis; the reduced expression of these interleukins due to the absence of stroma may have made the tumor less aggressive. It is yet to be discovered that these cases represent a new morphological spindle cell variant of DSRCT or new tumors sharing the same molecular genetics change. According to the author if these tumors are considered as morphological variants of DSRCT then their favorable clinical outcome is worth high lighting in the literature. The alternative characterization of these tumors is leimyosoarcoma with t (11; 22) (p13; q12). This lead us to speculate that there may be a separate group of spindle cell tumors in pediatric age group with leiomyosarcoma like morphology with cytokeratin expression having same translocation of DSRCT.

# Chapter V

# Immunohistochemical Findings

The immunohistochemical profile of DSRCT is considered a more reliable indicator of the tumor, by some authors, than the variable histologic pattern. Tumor cells show immunohistochemical reactivity for epithelial markers [cytokeratin, (Figure 9) epithelial membrane antigen (EMA)], muscle marker (desmin), (Figure 10) and mesenchymal marker (vimentin), (Figure 11). They show variable positivity for neural markers [CD 56, neuron-specific enolase (NSE)], The cellular stroma is immunoreactive for vimentin and muscle-specific actin. Variations of the typical phenotype have been reported, with some cases that are negative or that show only weak or focal positivity for several of these antibodies. Lack of keratin, desmin and NSE expression is also documented in 10-20% cases [76, 80]. Immunohistochemical variations include expression for FLI-1, CA-125, BER-EP4, ASMA, muscle specific actin, synaptophysin, chromogranin and CD 99 (Mic 2) expression [77].

According to the two comprehensive series by Ordonez and Gerald [10,76], tumor cells are consistently immunopositive for cytokeratin (86-95%), Epithelial membrane antigen EMA (93-96%), desmin (90-91%), vimentin (81-97%) and neuron specific enolase (72-81%), alpha smooth muscle actin (14-19%) and CD 99 MIC-2 in (20-30%) of cases.

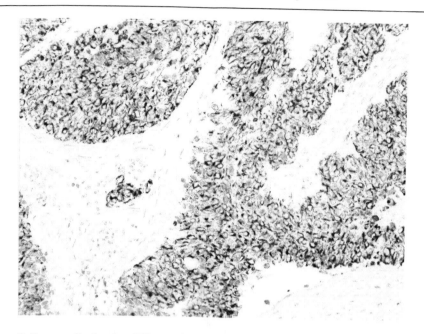

Figure 9: Tumor cells showing diffuse and strong immunoreactivity to cytokeratin. (Original magnification 200 x).

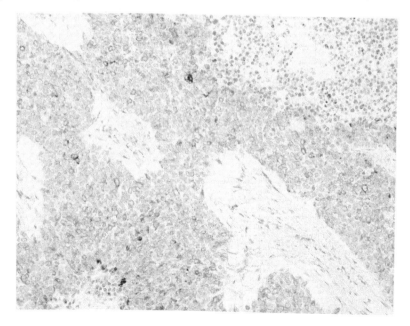

Figure 10: Dot like paranuclear desmin positivity. (Original magnification 200 x).

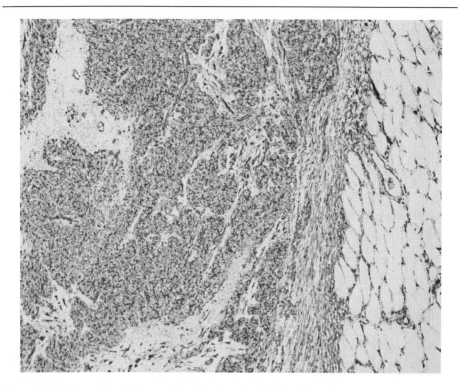

Figure 11: Tumor cells staining positive for vimentin. (Original magnification 200x).

The keratin positivity reported by Lae [80] in a review of 32 cases is 87% which was equal to what was reported by Gerald et al (86%) however lower than that reported by Ordonez et al (95%). Ordonez reported cytokeratin expression in 37(95%) of 39 cases when AE1/AE3/Cam 5.2 cocktail of anticytokeratin antibodies was used. The staining pattern was diffuse cytoplasmic; however dot like pattern of reactivity was seen in four tumors. Cytokeratin 20 and cytokeratin 5/6 was consistently negative in their study. EMA was positive in 24 out of 25 cases stained for this antibody and they included two cases which were negative for cytokeratins; therefore EMA appeared to be a more sensitive marker for the detection of epithelial differentiation when cytokeratin expression failed [76]. The pattern of staining for EMA was cytoplasmic. Gerald and Rosai reported reactivity for EMA in 21 of 21 cases. Among other epithelial markers MOC-31 positivity was reported by Ordonez et al in (90%) cases and Ber EP4 in 71% cases.

Immunostaining for desmin shows a distinct punctate and perinuclear cytoplasmic dot-like positivity as originally described by Gerald et al in more than half of the reported cases. Lae et al [80] has reported 81% desmin positivity as compared to 91% reported by Ordonez et al and 90% reported by Gerald et al in two large series. The co-expression of epithelial and mesenchymal intermediate filaments has also been reported in normal endometrium as well as in epithelial malignancies of uterus, ovary, kidney, lung and mesothelium. Coexpression of keratin, desmin, and vimentin has been reported in serous, pleural, and pericardial mesothelial cells as well as in normal smooth muscle cells and in smooth muscle and skeletal muscle neoplasms [73]. The presence of this intermediate filament suggests not only mesenchymal differentiation of this tumor but also suggests that it may originate from mesothelial or sub-mesothelial cells. Few IHC stains are consistently negative in DSRCT like markers of muscle differentiation (myogenin and Myo D1). No reactivity for MyoD1, myogenin and myoglobin was seen in the series presented by Ordonez [76]. Some of the reported cases have also shown positivity for S-100, Leu M1, glial fibrillary acidic protein, Leu7 and actin [73, 78,120]. Despite desmin reactivity stains for actin are only rarely and focally positive. The presence of desmin without convincing actin reactivity is probably not sufficient to indicate true myogenous differentiation. Actin positivity reported by Lae is 3%, which is similar to that reported by Gerald et al (2%) but lower than that reported by Ordonez (9%).

Cytoplasmic staining for CD99 (Mic-2) can also be seen. Besides Ewings sarcoma, DSRCT is one of two other sarcomas (the other being synovial sarcoma) that demonstrates CD99 (Mic-2) Positivity, but the staining pattern is usually cytoplasmic, as compared to the membranous staining seen in Ewings sarcoma / PNET [76,79]. CD99 positivity is reported 23% by Lae which is similar to that reported by Gerald et al (20%) but higher than that reported by Ordonez (12%).

CD117 is generally negative. None of the 8 DSRCT showed positivity for C-Kit in a study conducted by Smithey et al [79] to see c-Kit expression in pediatric solid tumors. Membrane positivity for CA 125 has also been described by Ordonez [68]. Reactivity for GFAP and neurofilament has not been reported in DSRCT [73].

It is debatable that DSRCT shows neural differentiation. Strong positivity for NSE is generally considered as the strongest evidence for neural differentiation, though NSE is known to be non-specific and shows reactivity in non-neuroendocrine and non-neural tumors of breast, lung, kidney and ovary [73]. According to Ordonez [71] 6 of 12 cases reacted for NSE, 2 of 11 cases for synaptophysin and none of 17 stained for chromogranin A. Similar results were reported by Gerald et al [2] 4 of 8 tumors stained for NSE, and none of the 8 cases stained for chromogranin A or the one for synaptophysin showed reactivity for either of these markers. The results for Neuron specific enolase reported by Lae et al (84%) are similar to those reported by Gerald et al and Ordonez.

Cases have been described in the literature that lacked immune-histochemical evidence of epithelial differentiation, but were found to have the fusion transcripts characteristic of DSRCT. Trupiano et al [81] has described two patients (a 41-year-old male and a 31-year-old female) who presented with large intra abdominal masses. Histology was consistent with a DSRCT, however, immunohistochemically neither case expressed any of the epithelial markers including AE1/AE3, CAM 5.2 and EMA, however, were immunoreactive for vimentin, and desmin, including one which had the characteristic dot-like pattern of immunoreactivity. Zhang et al [74] also reported a case of DSRCT with atypical morphological features comprising of microcystic areas and anastomosing trabeculae and cords with abundant myxoid stroma and prominent endothelial proliferation. The tumor cells were positive for desmin and vimentin however were negative for multiple epithelial markers including pan-cytokeratin, CAM 5.2, cytokeratins 7 & 20 and epithelial membrane antigen. These cases clearly emphasize the need for molecular confirmation with ambiguous morphological and immunohisto-chemical features.

Nishio et al [82] has described an adult case of intra abdominal small round cell tumor that possessed t (11; 22) (p13; q12) translocation detected by RT-PCR but that lacked desmoplasia and immunohistochemical evidence of epithelial differentiation. The author questioned that the identification of the t (11; 22) (p13; q12) translocation by RT-PCR should be taken as absolute proof of a diagnosis of DSRCT in the absence of typical histological and immunophenotypic features.

The WT1 gene is located at 11p13, and its product is a 52- to 54-kD nuclear protein that has four zinc fingers and acts as a transcriptional regulator, mainly as a repressor. Mutations affecting the zinc finger regions abolish this function. WT1 is transcribed in various tissues including kidney, gonads, uterus, brain, mesothelium, and spleen and its expression has also been reported in various tumors as melanoma, mesothelioma, human acute leukemias, and to a lesser degree in epithelial ovarian tumors [82]. In DSRCT, by analogy with other ES fusion products, the EWS-WT1 chimera would have the potential to promote tumorigenesis by acting as an aberrant transcription factor [82]. Barnoud et al [83] has shown in his study that WT1 is a sensitive and specific marker for DSRCT and can be used to differentiate it from other small round cell tumors. Immunohistochemistry for WT 1 using antibodies to both terminals should provide a useful test to demonstrate EWS-WT 1 fusion transcript of DSRCT that encodes the C- terminal but not the N- terminal of WT 1. DSRCT should be positive for the C- terminal antibody but negative for the N- terminal antibody. Other tumors like rhabdoid tumor, mesothelioma and Wilms tumor that express wild type WT 1 should be positive for both antibodies, and tumors that do not express wild type WT 1 should be negative for both antibodies. Murphy et al [16] reported positive nuclear staining for WT 1 C- terminal antibody and lack of nuclear staining for for WT 1 N- terminal in 83% cases of DSRCT. Other studies showed positive staining for WT 1 C- terminal in 90% of DSRCT and absence of nuclear staining for WT 1 N- terminal antibodyin 98% cases. Wang et al [33] reported positive cytoplasmic staining for the N- terminal antibody and concluded that both antibodies could come positive in DSRCT and therefore it is not useful in identifying the characteristic translocation. Barnoud et al [83] reported immunohistochemical expression of WT1 in 15 patients having DSRCT. WT (C-19) immunoreactivity was present in all 15 cases (100%) of DSRCT. 11 cases showed diffuse nuclear reactivity (3+), while 4 cases showed 2 + nuclear positivity. 3 cases showed diffuse weak to moderate cytoplasmic positivity. They emphasized on the use of C- terminal antibody alone in distinguishing DSRCT from other small round cell tumors. In different studies almost all

DSRCT are positive for WT1 [84, 85]. Hill et al [84] studied the predictive value of immunohistochemistry with an antibody to the C- terminal region of the Wilms tumor (WT1) protein for differentiating DSRCT or EWS/PNET in 24 malignant small round cell tumors that were previously diagnosed as DSRCT or EWS/PNET by standard methods. In their study, 6 out of 13 cases of DSRCT were confirmed by RT-PCR and all six cases showed EWS-WT1 fusion and all 13 DSRCTs showed strong definitive nuclear staining with the WT1 antibody. According to his study, WT1 antibody staining predicts the EWS-WT1 translocation with high sensitivity and specificity and was found to be useful in differentiating DSRCT from EWS-PNET when genetic information is not available.

Ordonez also showed WT1 part of the chimeric protein produced by the translocation t (11; 22) detected by immunohistochemistry using antibody raised against the carboxy terminal of WT1. This strong nuclear staining could represent accumulation of the protein as a result of hybrid gene expression. Lae et al showed 91% positivity for WT1, with cells showing weak and focal nuclear staining and fairly constant paranuclear cytoplasmic staining.

Murphy et al [16] have reported a new molecular variant of soft tissue DSRCT in a 15-year-old-male. The tumor was negative for the WT1 C-terminal and showed nuclear staining with the N-terminal antibody. This case also demonstrated 2 novel fusion transcripts, both lacking WT1 exons 9 and 10 and one containing additional exons of WT1 (exons3-7). The tumor strongly expressed full length WT1 and showed negative staining for the WT1 C-terminus and positive nuclear staining with the N-terminal antibody. This was a paradoxical staining pattern of WT1 in DSRCT associated with 2 highly unusual variant transcripts suggesting that the immunostaining pattern may be altered by variant transcripts.

The EWS-WT1 fusion encodes a novel transcription factor comprising a strong EWS transcriptional activation domain merged with a WT1 DNA binding domain. This fusion creates an oncogenic chimaera, which may lead to loss of the tumor suppressor effects of the WT1 gene, in addition to an increase in the EWS driven expression of growth factors usually repressed by WT1. WT1 is reported to regulate connective tissue growth factor (CCN2) expression via novel elements in the promoter region of CCN2. Rachfal et al

[151] stated that DSRCT expresses CCN2 in the tumor cells as well as in the supporting stromal fibroblasts and vascular endothelial cells, suggesting that CCN2 may play a role in autocrine and paracrine regulation of tumor cell growth, matrigenesis, and angiogenesis. CCN2 and other CCN proteins can be useful targets for novel therapeutic approaches for treating DSRCT.

# Chapter VI

# Cytological Features

The literature on cytological features of DSRCT including needle aspirates and ascetic and pleural fluids is limited and includes only handful of reports. The typical cytology of DSRCT was first described by Setrakian et al [87] who studied Fine needle aspiration biopsy (FNAB) of masses and metastases in pleural and ascetic body fluids and in conventional smears and thin prep samples. Cytologically, the smears are moderately cellular and the tumor cells are arranged mostly in loose clusters or lie singly. The tumor clusters occasionally are organized in sheets, three-dimensional groups, or tissue fragments and consist of small, round to oval cells with a scant amount of light blue or purple cytoplasm which is scanty to moderate with variable number of vacuoles. Cells have high nuclear-cytoplasmic ratios containing granular chromatin. The nuclei are round to oval with fine granular chromatin pattern and nucleoli are inconspicuous or absent [87, 88, 89]. Some authors have noted prominent nucleoli [90, 91]. Necrosis has also been reported in cytology samples. Mitotic figures are rare. Analysis is possible from tissue biopsy and FNA specimens as well as ascitic and pleural tap fluid. Effusion samples show similar cytological features with cohesive cell clusters. Nuclear molding and individual necrotic cells may be present. Occasionally spindle fibroblast like cells are sometimes observed [94]. The hypocellular stromal fragments appear pink to metachromatic on Diff Quick and May-Grunwald-Giemsa stains and pale blue on Papanicolau technique.

Granja et al [92] have studied cytological features of one FNAB sample and three from serous effusions (2 peritoneal fluid samples and one pleural effusion sample). All smears showed high cellularity. Nuceli were round to oval with small nucleoli. Tumor cells were clustered and rare clusters showed rosette like features in FNAB sample. However, the tumor cells in effusion samples were more frequently arranged in three dimensional clusters and rosettes were rarely observed. No fragments of fibrosis, cytoplasmic granules or vacuoles were seen. The finding of stromal fragments which is a frequent finding in FNA is not a common finding in liquid base preparations [96].

Dave et al [93] reported fine needle aspiration biopsy (FNAB) findings in seven aspirates from four cases of histologically and immunohistochemically confirmed cases. One case showed pseudorosette like structures and two cases showed small tubules. The nuclei showed finely granular chromatin with grooves, infoldings/lobulations of nuclear membranes, nuclear molding and inconspicuous nucleoli. Stromal fragments were noted in all four cases. These stromal fragments were hypocellular and contained few fibroblasts. Tumor cells were seen trapped in the stroma. No necrosis was seen in any case. In their study, it was found that although cytology is not the gold standard of diagnosis but coupled with immunocytochemistry can serve as a mode of pre-operative diagnosis where biopsy is difficult to obtain.

Akhtar et al [94] has described clusters of rounded tumor cells accompanied by larger fragments of stroma. In areas individual cells or small group of cells separated by small amount of intercellular stroma were seen. Most of the tumor cells showed cytoplasmic vacuoles and in some cells the entire cytoplasm was replaced by vacuoles.

Presley et al [95] evaluated the cytologic preparation for cellularity, cohesion, cell architecture, cell size, nuclear features (presence of nucleoli, chromatin pattern), molding, nuclear to cytoplasmic (N: C) ratio, cytoplasmic characteristics, stroma, DNA streaking, mitoses, apoptosis and background histiocytes, and reported differences between the postchemotherapy and prechemotherapy specimens. The initial smears showed cellular aspirates with high N: C ratio. Irregular nuclear membrane clefts, finely granular chromatin and a variable degree of DNA streaking, molding, mitoses, and metachromatic stroma. The most striking postchemotherapy change seen in the smears was prominent nucleoli, along with predominantly discohesive single cell architecture, absence of mitotic figures, more abundant stroma and large cell size.

Crapanzano et al [96] have reported cytological features in five aspirates and two ascitic fluid samples including the direct smears and the thin Prep specimens. All specimens were moderate to highly cellular and contained single cells and cell clusters, fine to moderately granular chromatin, nuclear molding and hypocellular stroma. One case showed hypercellular stroma. Stromal fragments were present in the direct smears but were uncommon in thin Prep. Three of the five thin Prep specimens and all the direct smears demonstrated three-dimensional cell groups. Pseudorosettes were noted in all cases except one. No true glands with central lumina were seen. Cytoplasmic vacuoles were also a constant feature except in one case in which rare vacuoles were seen. A notable feature in one specimen of ascetic fluid was the presence of occasional tumor cells arranged in a single-file pattern reminiscent of invasive lobular carcinoma of breast.

Recently it is reported in the left submandibular gland [97], which is a rare location, diagnosed by FNAC showed variably cohesive clusters of small basaloid cells with hyperchromatic nuclei and fine granular chromatin. It should be considered in the differential diagnosis of a salivary gland neoplasm with a basaloid or small cell pattern on fine-needle aspiration cytology.

Review of literature suggests that cytological diagnosis is plausible and in conjunction with immunocytochemistry may help in documenting the polyphenotypic nature and thereby confirming the diagnosis.

# Chapter VII

# Radiographic Features

The clinical features of DSRCT are sufficient to warrant sonographic and cross sectional imaging evaluation. In this context, multi-detector computerized tomographic scan has valuable role. The radiological features of this tumor have been reported initially by case reports [98]. Because of the often nonspecific manifestations, patients are often referred for cross-sectional imaging.

## Plain X-Ray Features

The plain X-ray abdomen is not helpful because of the diverse nonspecific presentation of abdominal symptoms. It may show non specific finding of increased radiographic opacity with displacement of adjacent bowel or viscera depending upon the size and location of the mass. This finding although non-specific or incidental may be a stepping stone for further evaluation. Furthermore, other associated findings such as generalized haziness as seen in ascites or air fluid levels as seen in intestinal obstruction could be detected.

# Ultrasonography

Ultasonography is a non invasive, easily available and relatively cheap imaging tool to show these tumors provided their location and size is favorable with proficiency of the sonographer. Ultrasonographically, the tumors have defined borders and are of hypoechoic echotexture without evidence of increased through- transmission reflecting their solid nature. In addition to good access to abdominal viscera, other ancillary findings like free intraperitoneal fluid, para aortic lymphadenopathy and pleural effusion can be assessed. In patients with large amount of ascites, ultrasound is capable of demonstrating superficial peritoneal and omental tumor nodules as small as 2 to 3 mm because of the acoustic window provided by the peritoneal fluid. However, it is difficult to detect peritoneal masses in patients with little or no ascites. Furthermore, centrally located tumors are poorly imaged by ultrasound due to the acoustic impedance of bowel gas and mesenteric fat.

# Computerized Tomography

Computerized tomogram (CT) scanning is the most commonly utilized and useful diagnostic modality. DSRCT are often evaluated with cross-sectional imaging [99]. Now with the use of multidetector CT scanners, lesions less than 1 cm in diameter can be detected before they are large enough to cause symptoms. Careful attention to technique is important in detecting small intraperitoneal soft tissue masses of non-visceral origin. It is particularly important to opacify the GI tract with oral contrast material so that unopacified bowel is not mistaken for a mesenteric mass. Conversely, a small mesenteric mass can be obscured if surrounded by unopacified bowel loops. If bowel cannot confidently be distinguished from a mesenteric mass, additional contiguous scans through the suspicious area can be obtained after additional oral contrast material has been administered or after delay allows transit of more proximal contrast material. Occasionally, it is helpful to opacify the colon per rectum with a dilute contrast solution or air in order to differentiate a redundant sigmoid colon from a pelvic mass. Furthermore, reading the images with thin slices reconstruction and multiplanar reformatting on work-stations is of immense aid. Intraperitoneal air or iodinated contrast material may improve the detection of implants in some intraperitoneal compartments [100].

CT scan reveals evidence of disseminated intra abdominal malignancy and mesothelial like growth pattern with extensive spread along the surface of the peritoneal cavity. Bulky heterogeneous peritoneal soft tissue masses without an apparent organ based primary are characteristic of DSRCT. Tumors often show inhomogeneous attenuation on CT.

Nowadays with the use of Multi-Detector CT (MDCT) scanner, ability to detect and characterize DSRCT has been found to high level of confidence, especially when studied with thin slices reconstruction and multiplanar reformatting on work-station. The masses are characteristically multilobulated in appearances and are heterogeneous in CT attenuation or have centrally located low-attenuation regions. Areas of central low attenuation on CT scans seem to correspond to focal hemorrhage or necrosis within the tumor on gross pathologic analysis. The tumor masses may contain small, punctate calcifications, visible readily on CT scans. Malignant ascites is frequently present. Complications such as bowel obstruction or ureteral obstruction may occur. The latter is particularly common in patients with dominant pelvic masses [102]. Mesenteric abnormalities are readily identified on CT in all but the leanest patients because of the abundance of fat present within the normal mesentery. Various pathologic processes, both benign and malignant, may infiltrate the mesentery causing an increase in attenuation of the mesenteric fat, distortion of the mesenteric architecture, and loss of definition of the mesenteric vessels. Some of these processes may also cause thickening of the peritoneal lining. Detection of mesenteric abnormalities requires rigorous attention to CT technique.

Pickhardt et al [101] described the abdominal CT findings very precisely in his retrospective study of 14 patients. The most characteristic imaging finding in DSRCT was multiple bulky peritoneal soft-tissue masses without an apparent organ-based primary site. The mean diameter of the masses was 5cm (range, 2-12cm), and there was a mean of 4.4 masses per case (range 1-17).

The tumors were predominantly intraperitoneal, with paravesical and omental sites. Areas of central low attenuation within the tumors, suggestive of hemorrhage or necrosis were seen in78% of the cases. The degree of tumor enhancement with intravenous contrast material was modest, approximately equal in attenuation to that of the abdominal wall musculature. Small foci of punctate calcification were present within tumors in 2 cases (22%). A retroperitoneal tumor was present in 3 patients (33%). Multiple rounded, hypo attenuating hepatic lesions were seen up to 5.5cm in diameter in 3 patients (33%). In addition to parenchymal hepatic metastases, CT also showed serosal tumor implants from intraperitoneal spread in 1 patient. Small to moderate amount of ascites was present in 5 patients (56%). Hypoattenuating abdominal or retroperitoneal lymphadenopathy was seen in 2 patients (22%). Hydronephrosis due to mass effect from a retroperitoneal tumor was detected in 2 patients (22%). The masses can present with moderately dilated bowel loops, a finding suggestive of partial obstruction by a tumor was found in 1 patient (11%).

The tumor spreads diffusely throughout the peritoneal surfaces therefore the primary imaging finding is the presence of peritoneal thickening, nodules, and masses. However, a solitary peritoneal mass may be the only finding seen at initial presentation [101]. Intraperitoneal primary masses may be large and bulky [102,103]. The majority of patients in the series reported by Bellah et al [102] had a dominant tumor mass larger than 10 cm. Egloff et al [35] has described Sonographic and multiphase CT findings in a renal DSRCT. Sonographic examination showed 5-cm well circumscribed heterogeneous mass in the mid portion of the left kidney, accompanied by small foci of punctate calcifications. On the unenhanced images of the CT, the mass was slightly hyperdense compared with the normal renal parenchyma and showed multiple foci of punctate calcifications. On the enhanced images of the CT, the mass was hypovascular and hypodense compared with the adjacent normally enhancing renal parenchyma. The punctate calcifications may be helpful in differentiating DSRCT from other common pediatric renal malignancies for example clear cell sarcoma and rhabdoid tumor lack calcifications. Calcifications seen in 5-15% of Wilms tumor are curvilinear rather than punctuate. Renal cell carcinomas are hypervascular as compared to the hypovascular DSRCT described by Egloff.

# Magnetic Resonance Imaging

Although CT remains the imaging method of choice for detecting these tumors, newer MRI techniques, including breath-hold gradient echo imaging with fat suppression and gadolinium enhancement, show promising results for demonstrating peritoneal based tumors. However, non-breath-hold MRI techniques suffer from image degradation due to motion artifact from respiration, cardiac activity, and bowel peristalsis, and from lack of a satisfactory GI contrast agent. Detection of implants by MRI is improved in the presence of ascites, with greatest contrast achieved on T1-weighted images obtained with fat suppression and gadolinium enhancement.

At MR imaging, the tumors are typically heterogeneous in signal intensity but predominantly hypointense with T1-weighted sequences and hyperintense with T2-weighted sequences [104,105]. Imaging after intravenous administration of gadolinium with fat suppression shows heterogeneous enhancement. Careful attention should be paid to all bones, solid organs, and lymphatic structures because hematogenous and lymphatic metastases are common at initial presentation as well as during disease progression. Fifty percent of the cases reported by Quaglia and Brennan [136] had distant metastasis at the time of presentation. Hematogenous metastasis to the liver, lung, and bone may occur. Magnetic resonance imaging is not as valuable as CT for detecting, characterizing, and delineating mesenteric abnormalities. Peristaltic and respiratory motion artifacts can degrade MR images and limit spatial resolution in the region of the mesentery. In addition, lack of a reliable oral contrast agent for MRI makes it difficult to differentiate mesenteric masses from bowel loops in many cases. Hence MRI appearance of nodular or thickened, enhancing peritoneum is a nonspecific finding, with considerable overlap between benign and malignant causes.

The main radiological features of the two cases presented by Outwater et al [97]were dominant well-defined tumor mass without obvious visceral organ origin and the tumors occurring in intra peritoneal location (i.e. the right paracolic gutter and retrovesical space) with evidence of multiple small peritoneal implants. Both tumors showed necrosis, with hemorrhagic necrosis evident on T1-weighted images in one tumor. Later on cross sectional imaging studies characterized these tumors typically as multiple, lobulated, peritoneal-based masses without an apparent organ of origin. Studies show that the paravesical region along with the omentum, are the most common sites of tumor involvement [99].

# Positron Emmission Tomography

Positron Emission Tomography using F-18 fluorodeoxyglucose can be a useful adjunct in the preoperative evaluation of soft tissue tumors and provide valuable information that cannot be obtained from CT or MRI. The whole body F-18 fluorodeoxyglucose positron emission tomography study shows multiple foci of increased metabolic activity in the abdomen and pelvis during or after multimodality therapy. It also helps in evaluation of post therapy recurrence of these tumors [106].

# Chapter VIII

# Differential Diagnosis

DSRCT should be considered in the differential diagnosis of a young male patient presenting with single or multiple peritoneal masses. The radiologic differential diagnosis for multiple solid peritoneal masses is broad and includes various neoplastic, inflammatory, and miscellaneous processes. Radiological differential diagnosis in case of solitary large intra-peritoneal mass includes desmoid tumor, peritoneal mesothelioma and malignant fibrous histiocytoma. Differential diagnosis in cases of huge intra- and retroperitoneal mass with or without seeding includes neuroblastoma, germ-cell tumor, wilms' tumor, desmoid tumor and Ewings sarcoma/PNET. Differential diagnosis for diffuse intra peritoneal nodules or masses includes peritoneal lymphomatosis, intraperitoneal rhabdomyosarcoma, peritoneal mesothelioma, and even secondary seeding of intracranial tumors by ventriculoperitoneal shunts. When peritoneal masses are discovered, the principal diagnostic concern is metastatic disease, which is the most frequently encountered neoplastic process that involves the peritoneal cavity. However, primary peritoneal tumors should be included in the differential diagnosis, particularly when there is no evidence of a primary visceral malignancy. DSRCT should be included in the differential diagnosis of widespread peritoneal malignant disease on radiologic examination.

Peritoneal carcinomatosis from a variety of primary malignancies, including ovarian, gastrointestinal, and lymphomatous sources, may manifest as solid masses or infiltration of the intraabdominal fat. It occurs in relatively older age group. Sarcomatosis usually presents as a dominant mesenteric, pelvic or small bowel closely related mass with bulky necrotic tumors along peritoneal or mesenteric surfaces. Sarcomatosis often lacks ascites and has extensive liver metastases. Malignant mesothelioma of the peritoneum is usually infiltrative but may also manifest as discrete tumors, which are usually accompanied by a variable amount of ascites. Gastrointestinal carcinoid, malignant melanoma, and soft-tissue sarcomas such as malignant fibrous histiocytoma may also have a similar radiologic appearance [105]. Desmoid fibromatosis, peritoneal tuberculosis, fibrosing mesenteritis, splenosis, and amyloidosis are other disorders whose infiltrative and/or tumefactive manifestations overlap with the appearance of desmoplastic small round cell tumor [106,107]. The omental and mesenteric masses of desmoplastic small round cell tumor may resemble conditions with marked lymphadenopathy, such as malignant lymphoma, Castleman's disease, Whipple disease, mycobacteriosis, actinomycosis, and other conditions with bulky intraabdominal disease [108,109,110]. Retroperitoneal lymphadenopathy appears to be less extensive in desmoplastic small round cell tumor than in lymphoma. When soft-tissue masses are confined to the pelvis in female patients, a neoplastic or inflammatory disorder of the reproductive tract is a reasonable initial consideration. Leiomyomatosis peritonealis disseminata, a rare condition affecting premenopausal women, can appear similar to desmoplastic small round cell tumor at imaging [111]. Likewise, with a scrotal mass in a young male patient, diagnostic considerations include germ cell and other testicular neoplasms, paratesticular sarcoma, and tumefactive inflammatory processes. The paratesticular location of desmoplastic small round cell tumor allows exclusion of the much more common testicular neoplasms.

In practice, the presence of a presumed organ-based primary site strongly favors the diagnosis of carcinomatosis, whereas an associated pleural rind likely represents mesothelioma. In the absence of an apparent primary tumor in an adolescent or young adult, desmoplastic small round cell tumor should be considered in the differential diagnosis. Tumor hemorrhage or necrosis and ascites can be seen with most of the aforementioned entities but are more common with malignancies, tuberculous peritonitis, and desmoplastic small round cell tumor. A patient age of less than 25 years might favor the diagnosis of desmoplastic small round cell tumor or inflammatory diseases. However, given the large overlap in the radiologic appearances of peritoneal diseases, histological evaluation is generally recommended.

Primary neoplasms of the peritoneum are generally of mesenchymal origin. Desmoid tumors are often associated with Gardner's syndrome which usually occurs in the adult population with female predominance and they lack ascites. The mesenteric desmoid tumor is a non-encapsulated, locally invasive form of fibromatosis. It occurs predominantly in patients with Gardner's syndrome who have undergone abdominal surgery, although it sometimes occurs as an isolated abnormality. On CT scan, a desmoid tumor appears as a soft tissue mass displacing adjacent visceral structures. Although the mass may appear well circumscribed, it often has irregular margins reflecting its infiltrative nature. Other neoplasms such as mesenteric metastases and lymphoma can have a similar appearance on CT scan. On MRI a desmoid tumor appears low in signal intensity on T1-weighted images and remains relatively low in intensity on T2-weighted images, reflecting its large fibrous composition.

Peritoneal lymphomatosis often has a more infiltrative appearance and is usually accompanied by retroperitoneal lymphadenopathy and lacks ascites and areas of necrosis.

Lipomatous tumors, which occur predominantly in the retroperitoneum, rarely involve the peritoneal cavity. Benign lipomas consist predominantly of fat, which is reflected in their CT attenuation and MR signal characteristics. Multiple histologic subtypes of liposarcoma exist, each with corresponding CT and MR characteristics. Well-differentiated liposarcoma can be of lipomatous or sclerosing type, with CT and MR appearance of fat or muscle, respectively. Myxoid liposarcoma has an appearance on unenhanced CT that is similar to water, with reticular enhancement after administration of intravenous contrast material. Round cell and pleomorphic liposarcomas are nonfatty tumors with nonspecific soft tissue appearance on CT and MRI.

Benign or malignant primary peritoneal tumors other than desmoid and lipomatous tumors are rare but can arise from any of the mesenchymal tissue elements. Primary mesenteric and omental teratomas have also been reported. Because both benign and malignant primary peritoneal tumors may demonstrate cystic, solid, and complex features, histologic diagnosis is usually required.

Mesothelioma is a rare malignant neoplasm arising from the serosal lining of the pleura, peritoneum, and pericardium. Peritoneal involvement may occur, either alone or in combination with pleural involvement. CT findings in patients with peritoneal mesothelioma include peritoneal thickening that may appear irregular or nodular, omental and mesenteric thickening, and ascites. It can also appear as a multilocular cystic mass. The mesenteric involvement may produce a "stellate" appearance due to thickening of the perivascular bundles by tumor. The CT appearance of peritoneal mesothelioma may be indistinguishable from peritoneal carcinomatosis, lymphoma, and benign disease processes such as tuberculous peritonitis. The amount of ascites relative to the soft tissue component of mesothelioma may be disproportionately small as compared with peritoneal carcinomatosis in which ascites is usually a prominent feature.

The histopathologic differential diagnosis for DSRCT is influenced to some extent by the age of the patient at presentation. The differential diagnosis in a child or adolescent includes rhabdomyosarcoma, non-Hodgkin lymphoma, Ewing sarcoma/primitive neuroectodermal tumor, blastemic Wilms tumor, neuroblastoma, anaplastic synovial sarcoma, ectomesenchymoma. Immunohistochemical, electron microscopic, and molecular genetic studies allow reliable discrimination of these small cell neoplasms.

Differential diagnoses in adults include small cell carcinoma, lymphoma, poorly differentiated carcinoma, carcinoid tumor, merkle cell carcinoma, and malignant small cell mesothelioma. Similar histological features with these small round cell tumors poses differential diagnostic difficulties that necessitate the application of ancillary methods, such as immunohistochemistry and cytogenetic techniques.

The differential diagnosis in cases of IDSRCT involving the ovary is that of ovarian small cell carcinoma of hypercalcemic type (OSCCHT).

Histologically both tumors differ significantly. OSCCHT lacks the desmoplastic stroma characteristic of IDSRCT and when present it is diffuse and irregular in distribution. Also OSCCHT exhibits follicle like spaces lined by neoplastic cells and IDSRCT contains degenerative spaces that result from tumor necrosis. WT1 is characteristically positive in IDSRCT using an antibody against the C-terminal. OSCCHT is also usually WT1 positive but with an antibody against the N-terminal.

Differential diagnosis of pleural and pulmonary DSRCT includes small cell mesothelioma, Non-hodgkins' lymphoma and Ewing's sarcoma / PNET. The leading clinical differential diagnosis of DSRCT in a pleural location is malignant mesothelioma. However the cytological and morphological features of DSRCT differ from most types of mesotheliomas and the immune-histochemical profile of positive staining for Ber Ep4, B72.3 and Leu M1 also differs from the marker profile of mesothelioma. Closest differential diagnosis is small cell mesothelioma however electron microscopic features of DSRCT fails to demonstrate cytoplasmic microvillus like projections [88]. Small cell mesotheliomas occur in older patients (>60 years) with a history of asbestos exposure.

The differential diagnosis of intracranial DSRCT includes in addition to most of the small round blue cell tumors, classic medulloblastoma and desmoplastic medulloblastoma. Classic medulloblastoma lacks the desmoplastic stroma and the elongated (carrot-like) shape of the nuclei, and it immunehistochemically shows neuronal or glial differentiation, coupled with negativity for keratin and desmin. Desmoplastic medulloblastoma has abundant connective tissue but the IHC features are the same as for the classic medulloblastoma [26]. Yachnis et al [113] reported "desmoplastic primitive neuroectodermal tumor with divergent differentiation" in the posterior fossa of a 9-month old girl. This tumor had marked morphological resemblance to DSRCT in that it showed sharply demarcated nests of tumor cells separated by abundant cellular stroma. Immunohistochemically the tumor was positive for GFAP, neurofilament, and synaptophysin and was negative for desmin. It was interpreted as mixed mesenchymal and primitive neuroectodermal tumor. The tumor recurrence was substantially different because it showed epithelial like nests and clusters of neoplastic cells, including islands of neuropil-containing ganglion cells.

The main differential diagnosis of DSRCT in bone is Ewings sarcoma / primitive neuroectodermal tumor (ES/PNET). ES / PNET is characterized by solid, densely packed sheets of undifferentiated mesenchymal cells, with or without rosette formation, which usually express CD 99, FL-1, and vimentin, and may also express markers of neural and neuroendocrine differentiation (NSE, S-100, CD 56, GFAP, Leu-7, chromogranin, synaptophysin).

The differential diagnosis of DSRCT in kidney is broad and includes blastema predominant wilms' tumor, primitive neuroectodermal tumor, metastatic neuroblastoma, rhabdoid tumor, small cell carcinoma, clear cell carcinoma and lymphoma. The peak incidence of Wilms tumor and clear cell sarcoma of kidney is between 2 and 3 years, congenital mesoblastic nephromas and rhabdoid tumors during infancy and primitive neuro-ectodermal tumors during adolescence. All four renal DSRCT presented by Wang et al [33] occurred between 6 and 8 years which is not the peak age for presentation of other types of renal tumors having similar histologic appearance as DSRCT.

The differential diagnosis of DSRCT in para-testicular area includes rhabdomyosarcoma and lymphoma. Rhabdomyosarcoma, however, occurs at a younger age (mean, 6.6 years) than paratesticular DSRCT (mean, 28 years). Almost 25% of paratesticular rhabdomyosarcomas have spindle cell morphology, which is rarely seen in DSRCT [114].

Differential diagnosis of round blue cell tumors in sinonasal region is broad and includes olfactory neuroblastoma, sinonasal undifferentiated carcinoma, non-hodgkins lymphoma, Ewing's Sarcoma, Embryonal and alveolar rhabdomyosarcoma. Olfactory neuroblastoma has a lobular growth pattern however necrosis and desmoplastic stroma is not typically seen in it. They show strong positivity for neural markers and only one third are positive for low molecular weight keratins.

# Chapter IX

# Ultrastructural Features

Ultrastructurally, the tumor cells display a primitive appearance with scanty and poorly developed cell junctions. Ultrastructural features described by Gerald [2] include scanty non-descript cytoplasm, irregularly shaped nuclei, numerous ribosomes, few mitochondria and profiles of granular endoplasmic reticulum. Paranuclear aggregates and whorls of intermediate sized cytoplasmic filaments, consistent with the perinuclear dot like staining pattern of desmin on immunohistochemical staining were also described. Ordonez et al [76] studied ultrastructural features of 16 cases of DSRCT and found variation in different cases of these juxtanuclear cytoplasmic aggregates of intermediate filaments. They varied from small aggregates to large aggregates occupying major portion of cytoplasm. They were seen both in round and spindle shaped tumor cells. Ordonez [68, 71] described that the tumor was made of solid groups of neoplastic cells surrounded by thin basal lumina. Nuclei were elongated with irregular nuclear contours and nuclear infoldings. Small well circumscribed nucleoli were also seen.

Secretory lumina, desmosomes, cell processes with microtubules have also been described in literature. Rare dense core granules compatible with a neuroendocrine nature were also seen in some cases. Gerald et al [2] described it in only two out of 14 cases evaluated ultrastructurally. Tumor cells had rudimentary cell processes and lacked well formed microvilli. Few cells were connected by cell junction complexes, including well formed desmosomes. In some cases, intraluminal microvillus-like structures, polar cell processes, microtubules, lipid droplets, glycogen, and dense core granules have been reported [3]. Intracytopasmic droplets of lipid and moderate amount of glycogen was also reported in 5/16 and 3/16 cases respectively by Ordonez et al. Although microvilli were noted by ordonez, they were not reported by Gerald in his study of 19 cases. Most cells have a primitive / undifferentiated appearance with small amounts of cytoplasm and scant organelles.

Bian et al [88] have described indented round to oval nuclei with heterochromatin margination to the nuclear membrane and occasional prominent nucleoli along with abundant polyribosomes. Perinuclear whorl like collections of intermediate filaments and well developed desmosome like cell to cell junctions were also observed.

DSRCT of the pancreas reported by Bismar et al [42] showed irregular nuclear outline and clumped chromatin on ultra structural examination. Discontinuous basement membrane was noted and the cells were connected with rudimentary cell junctions. The cytoplasm contained scattered cytoplasmic organelles consistent with glycogen, mitochondria and rough endoplasmic reticulum. Perinuclear clusters of intermediate cytoplasmic filaments were also seen.

# Chapter X

# Cytogenetics

DSRCT is associated with a novel, specific chromosomal abnormality, t (11; 22) (p13; q12), involving the EWS gene on 22q12 and the WT1 gene on 11p13. This unique reciprocal translocation was identified in 1992 by Sawyer et al [117] and was subsequently confirmed by several other investigators [76,118,119]. The EWS-WT1 transcript occurs in 96- 97% of DSRCT and it has become the sine qua non condition for its diagnosis [76]. This trans-location and the resultant fusion transcript have not been described in any other tumor type. Cases lacking this translocation and showing only disruptions of the 22q12 and 11q13 regions have also been reported [119]. In an analysis of 49 tumors, including Peripheral primitive neuroectodermal tumors, Wilms' tumors and rhabdomyosarcomas, de Alava et al [120] were unable to detect the EWS-WT1 fusion transcript by RT-PCR in any tumor other than DSRCT.

This unique translocation has breakpoints involving two chromosomal regions previously implicated in other malignant developmental tumors. Band 22q12 is the site of EWS, a gene disrupted in several tumor specific chromosomal translocations and 11p13 is the site of the Wilms' tumor gene WT1. This gene fusion is postulated to produce an oncogenic chimeric protein with the zinc finger DNA- binding domains of WT1 with the transcriptional regulatory domain of the Ewing's sarcoma (EWS) gene [127,128,129, 132,

133,134]. The translocation leads to the fusion of exon 7 of Ewings' sarcoma gene EWS on chromosome 22 with exon 8 of Wilms' tumor suppressor gene WT1 on chromosome 11. The resulting fusion protein couples the EWS activation domain to the WT1 zinc finger DNA binding domain. The chimeric protein leads to an over expression of WT1 protein in the tumor cells. It can be detected with the WT1 (C19) antibody directed to the carboxy terminal of WT1 but cannot be detected with the WT1 antibody to the amino terminus of WT1. The chimeric mRNA is detectable by reverse-transcriptase polymerase chain reaction analysis, and the chimeric protein is detectable by immune-histochemistry. Reverse transcriptase-polymerase chain reaction reveals EWS-WT1 fusion transcripts.

The EWS gene is most frequently involved in translocations in Ewings sarcoma/PNET, clear cell sarcoma, DSRCT, extraskeletol myxoid chondro-sarcoma, and rare cases of myxoid liposarcomas. The EWS gene encodes a 656-amino-acid protein of unknown function with a putative RNA binding site similar to RNA polymerase II, and, is the gene most commonly involved in reciprocal sarcoma translocations. WT1 is a tumor suppressor gene expressed in the developing genitourinary tract and is mutated in about 10 % of wilms' tumors. It encodes a zinc finger transcription factor that acts as a transcriptional repressor in vitro and plays a fundamental role in development of the kidney and other mesodermally derived tissues. The chimeric protein produced by the t (11;22) (p13;q12) functions as a transcriptional active, for inducing production of endogenous platelet-derived growth factor (PDGF) amongst other tumorigenic stimuli.

The specific gene translocation in sarcomas can be detected by various methods including southern blot, fluorescent in situ hybridization (FISH) and reverse transcriptase-polymerase chain reaction (RT-PCR). PCR-based assays have been shown to accurately detect EWS-WT1 fusion mRNA in fresh tumor tissue of DSRCT [120]. RT-PCR is rapid, easy to perform, inexpensive, specific and has potential application to small tissue specimens, such as fine-needle aspirates [121]. Southern blot and FISH require fresh tissue sections however RT-PCR can also be used with formalin fixed and paraffin embedded tissue sections [80].

Fluorescense in situ hybridization using an EWS break apart probe cocktail can rapidly provide initial evidence for translocation involving the EWS locus, and direct EWS and WT1 fusion visualization may be accompanied using EWS and WT1 locus-specific probes. FISH assays may provide a viable rapid alternative to reverse transcriptase polymerase/chain reaction in the diagnosis of DSRCT.

Molecular variants of the EWS-WT1 gene fusion have been found in approximately 5% of the DSRCT. Most of the cases of DSRCT show EWS-WT-1 fusion transcript of the first 7 exons of the EWS gene and the last 3 exons (exon 8-10) of the WT-1 gene. The translocation produces in-frame fusion of exons 1 to 7 of the EWS gene and exons 8 to 10 of the WT1 gene. The resulting fusion protein couples the EWS activation domain to the WT1 zinc-finger DNA binding domain. Murphy et al [16] has described an unusual fusion transcript showing deletion of WT1 exons 9 and 10. 3 cases with variant transcript have been reported; all were soft tissue tumors with EWS-WT-1 9/8 variant transcripts [40,122,123]. Similar transcript has been seen in DSRCT of kidney [32]. It is difficult to establish an association between the site and specific transcript and difficult to comment on the prognostic implications. Two hybrid tumors with Ewings sarcoma/primitive neuroecto-dermal tumors and DSRCT features have been reported [124,125]. These tumors presented with clinical, morphological and immunophenotypic characteristics of DSRCT, but with a fusion transcript typical of ES/PNET: Reverse transcription polymerase chain reaction revealed in one case EWS-FL-1 fusion transcript and in the other case as EWS-ERG fusion transcript. Moreover, another ES/PNET feature in these two cases was the strong, membranous immunoreactivity for Mic2 protein. Ordi et al [124] reported this case of intra abdominal tumor in a young woman with clinical, morphologic and IHC features of DSRCT but with an EWS-ERG fusion transcript typical of ES/PNET. This transcript, associated with the t (21;22)(q22;q12) chromosomal translocation is found in approximately 5-10% of cases of ES/PNET rather than the more frequent EWS/FLI-1 fusion t(11;22)(q24;q12) to which it is closely related.

First unique case of hybrid tumor arising in the peritoneal cavity of a young male has been described by Katz et al [125]. On Reverse transcription polymerase chain reaction EWS/FLI-1 fusion transcript was found as seen in PNET/Ewing's sarcoma, instead of the EWS/WT1 transcript of DSRCT seen in intraabdominal round cell tumor in a young man with morphological features of both primitive neuroectodermal tumour (PNET) and intra-abdominal desmoplastic round cell tumour (DSRCT). Thorner et al reported an intra-abdominal tumor with clinical, histologic and immune-histochemical profile of DSRCT, which showed a EWS/FLI-1 chimeric transcript [126,127]. The existence of such a hybrid tumor in this location suggests that DSRCT and PNET may be related and possibly share a common histogenesis.

The EWS-WT1 fusion product has been shown to be able to transcriptionally activate insulin-like growth factor 1[128]. Werner et al [129] described a novel EWS/ WT1 gene fusion product, EWS-WT-1 5/10, in a six-year old boy having DSRCT. The novel EWS-WT-1 gene fusion product was able to stimulate expression of the insulin like growth factor-I receptor, a potent anti apoptotic receptor tyrosine kinase that may play an important role in DSRCT etiology.

The genetic pathogenesis resulting in DSRCT has not been fully elucidated. Like most oncogenic translocations, alteration of one allele of the EWS and WT1 genes is sufficient to induce tumorigenesis in abdominal DSRCT, however, 2 extra-serosal DSRCT in adults had 2 chimeric transcripts suggesting that EWS-WT1 haplo-insufficiency is inadequate to transform extra-serosal cells [32, 40]. This speculation also explains why extra-serosal DSRCT are so rare and why they occurred in older patients. Another explanation is molecular diversity caused by internal deletion, exon skipping, and random nucleotide insertions in the EWS gene [130].

A new human cell line JN-DSRCT-1 is the first permanent human DSRCT cell line. The JN-DSRCT-1 cell line established by Nishio et al [131] from the pleural effusion of a 7-year old boy with pulmonary metastases, exhibits the unique morphologic and genetic characteristics of DSRCT. JN-DSRCT-1 exhibited a small round shape with immunopositive reactions for epithelial, mesenchymal, and neural markers. It will provide a new experimental system for a variety of important studies such as identifying the pathogenic mechanism, biologic behavior, and therapeutic strategies and reagents against human DSRCT.

# Chapter XI

# **Treatment**

The treatment modalities and impact on survival have been studied in small number of cases and current literature suggests that available treatment options do not impart long-term survival benefits. DSRCT presents with a short duration of nonspecific symptoms and the disease is fatal regardless of the treatment modality with 3 year survival of less than 30% [135]. Treatment modalities include chemotherapy, surgical resection, radiotherapy followed by autologous bone marrow transplantation. The standard treatment protocol has not been well documented and because of heterogeneity of the therapeutic modalities utilized, it is difficult to compare the efficacy and effectiveness of various regimens.

Surgical resection is often technically feasible to remove large peritoneal masses using a tangential dissection technique. It is usually performed followed by three to four cycles of chemotherapy producing considerable shrinkage of the tumor and marked reduction of tumor vascularity. The goal of surgery is removal of all gross tumor with removal of intra-abdominal/ pelvic masses and serosal implants. Another important role of surgery is the symptomatic relief of gastrointestinal obstruction, which reportedly develops in half of the patients. It has been noticed that these tumors spread over peritoneal surface and only invade focally into the underlying viscera therefore good surgical resection with patience is required for complete surgical removal. Since abdominopelvic tumor sometimes invades /tightly adheres to the viscera, all patients receive mechanical and antibiotic bowel preparation prior to definitive resection. Tumor masses that invade deeply into the muscle layers can be removed by wedge resection preserving the length of bowel.

Complete surgical resection is rarely possible in extensive sub diaphragmatic disease involving liver parenchyma or hilum and diaphragm and with infiltration into hepatic veins and inferior vena cava. This reflects the invasive and metastatic potential of the tumor. In these cases La Quaglia and Brennen [136] from the Memorial Sloan-Kettering Cancer center have attempted aggressive surgical resection with removal of maximum tumor load followed by chemotherapy and stem cell transplant. Radiation therapy is then delivered to entire abdomen with increased dosage to sites of residual disease. It is correlated with a better outcome but has not resulted in long term disease free survival. La Quaglia recommend external beam radiotherapy after surgery and neo-adjuvant chemotherapy and reported 3-year survival of 29% in a series of 40 patients. Although this study reported improved survival at 3 and 5 years, the overall prognosis remains grim. Primary complete or partial removal of macroscopic disease was possible in 60% of patients in one series and was associated with a longer median survival [137]. Farhat et al [139] have expressed concern about the efficacy of radiation with the diffuse peritoneal involvement of this tumor and potential toxicity to adjacent viscera, particularly small bowel.

For paratesticular tumors, a radical inguinal orchiectomy should be done as initial procedure followed by neoadjuvant chemotherapy. Abdominal exploration and gross total resection of metastatic lymph nodes and the ipsilateral spermatic cord should be done after three to four cycles of chemotherapy [136]. Localized hepatic tumors are amenable to resection. Regional perfusion or infusion therapy to the liver is another possible approach as a supplement to standard chemotherapy [136].

Lal et al [138] reported surgical excision to be highly significant in a cohort of 66 patients. The 3-year survival was 58% in patients who underwent gross tumor resection as compared to 0% 3-year survival rate in patients with non-resectable tumor. They reported improved patient survival at 3 and 5 years treated with aggressive surgical resection of greater than 90% of extensive intra-abdominal neoplasm, P6 protocol and adjuvant radiotherapy.

DSRCT has been demonstrated to be a chemosensitive tumor, generally with short-lasting response and poor survival gain from systemic chemotherapy. Adjuvant chemotherapy is offered to almost all patients regardless of undergoing an optimal or a sub-optimal debulking because of tumors' high chemosensitivity. No consistent response to chemotherapy is seen in literature review. Farhat et al [139] recommended that PAVEP should be the first-line drug for treating DSRCT after review of 8 cases with complete remission from the treated 60 cases. However grade four neutropenia occurred in 69% cycles while administering PAVEP regimens despite prophylactic use of G-CSF in 90% of cases in his report. Due to uncertain therapeutic results and life threatening side effects of PAVEP, other safe and effective chemotherapeutic drugs should be considered. Gerald et al [2] reported a successful application of 5-FU in treating intra-abdominal DSRCT. Kretschmar et al [99] also reported 60% response rate to this tumor. 5-FU was applied instead of PAVEP regimen as the first line of drug due to myelosuppression and renal toxicity of PAVEP regimen.

Since DSRCT is sensitive to alkylating agents and is dose responsive, an intensive alkylator-based chemotherapy regimen appears to improve survival when compared with standard dose chemotherapy in retrospective series. Kushner et al [140] reported 3-year overall survival of 29% using the intensive alkylator based chemotherapy (P6 regimen) using cyclo-phosphamide, doxorubicin, vincristine alternating with ifosfamide and etoposide combined with other treatment modalities such as surgery, radiation, autologous stem cell rescue, or the combination of all of the above in 12 DSRCT patients. Systemic combination chemotherapy presented by Kurre et al [141] utilizing the intense alkylator therapy (P6 regimen) has been the cornerstone of initial treatment. The P6 protocol involves 7 courses of chemotherapy, courses 1-3 and 6 use cyclophosphamide, doxorubicin and vincristine. Courses 4, 5 and 7 are infusions of ifosfamide and etoposide. Debulking surgery is then attempted with a goal of at least 90% reduction of tumor bulk. P6 protocol improved progression free survival without significant survival benefit. Lal et al [138] reported four patients with no evidence of disease with extended long term follow-up treated with P6 protocol and tumor debulking. None of the patients in this series received radiotherapy. The P6 regimen consisted of cyclophosphamide 2100mg/mZ/d by 6-h IV infusion, on days 1 and 2 (total dose/cycle: 4200mg/m2) for cycles 1,2,4, and 6. In addition, doxorubicin, 75 mg/m2/d by 72-h IV infusion, and vincristine, 2 mg/m2 by 72-h IV infusion, are given beginning day 1 for cycles 1,2,4, and 6. This is followed by ifosfamide, 1800mg/mZ/d by 1-h IV infusion, and etoposide, 100mg/m2/d by 1-h IV infusion, given on days 1-5 for cycles 3, 5, and 7. Cycles start when the absolute neutrophil count is >500/gi and platelets >100k/lxI.

Gil et al [20] recommended performing perioperative intraperitoneal chemotherapy but no evidence of prolonged survival was observed. They reported that the median survival was 20 months in 4 patients with complete resection of tumors compared with 11 months in 3 patients without complete resection.

The European chemotherapy protocols reported by Bertuzzi et al [142] are equieffective, but are prescribed for four cycles, followed by similar management with surgery and radiotherapy. They reported the clinical and molecular results in 10 adult DSRCT prospectively treated by high-dose chemotherapy and autologous peripheral stem cell transplantation in conjunction with local treatment (surgery and/ or radiotherapy). After a median follow up of 35 months the median survival was 14 months. They suggested that high dose chemotherapy does not improve overall clinical results.

Aguilera et al [143] presented a case of a 5-year old child with high risk DSRCT with massive disseminated peritoneal implants who had complete response and sustained a remission for 21 months following therapy.

Abdominopelvic radiotherapy is recommended following debulking surgery and chemotherapy. Radiotherapy is most effective with minimal gross residual disease (< 2cm). Whole abdominopelvic irradiation (WAPI) has been reported by Goodman et al [144], as a novel approach for the residual disease following aggressive chemotherapy and debulking surgery. They studied 21 patients treated with combination chemotherapy and whole abdominopelvic irradiation (WAPI) with external beam radiation to the entire abdomen and pelvis at a dose of 30 Gy. The response was disappointing, with a median survival of 32 months and a median time to relapse of 19 months. The overall survival and relapse free survival rate reported by them at 3-years were 48% and 19% respectively. Their patients developed significant acute hematologic and gastrointestinal toxicity, medically, they all were managed successfully and completed their treatment course.

Buttle et al [145] suggested that patients presenting with early or peripheral disease with favorable radiological appearances and absence of metastases should be subjected to aggressive treatment course with a combination chemotherapy, surgical resection and local radiotherapy. However patients with non-resectable disease may be treated with palliative measures and surgical intervention should be undertaken for symptom relief. Palliative chemotherapy is controversial in this group and radiotherapy when used as an isolated treatment may impart more toxicity than benefit.

Newer therapeutic regimes include treatment specifically targeted against cellular regulatory mechanism of DSRCT. The fusion protein created by the characteristic chromosomal translocation, t(11,22)(p13,q12) has been shown to induce production of endogenous platelet derived growth factor (PDGF) [37], T cell acute lymphoblastic leukemia associated antigen 1 protein (TALLA-1) and interleukin -2/15. SU101, an inhibitor of the platelet derived growth factor (PDGF) receptor pathway, produced rapid symptomatic improvement and prolonged disease stabilization in a patient with refractory progressive DSRCT treated in a pediatric phase 1 trial [146]. Adamson et al [146] have reported progressive refractory DSRCT that responded to SU101 treatment with prolonged stabilization of the disease. However, a recent phase II trial of the tyrosine kinase inhibitor imatinib (Gleevec®) in relapsed pediatric tumors produced no responses in patients with DSRCT [147].

Mazuryk et al [148] has described the benefit of autologous stem cell support in this group of patients. Al Blushi et al [49] have shown the results of autologous BMT in 3 patients, 2 were in remission 2 and 6 years after initial diagnosis. Autologous BMT was favored by them in the care of patients whom had responded favorably to chemotherapy, surgical resection, and radiation therapy.

Immunotherapy approaches to DSRCT are also under investigation. The monoclonal antibody therapies used to target novel cell surface antigens expressed in human solid tumors are well described. Two antigens G (D2) and the antigen to antibody 8H9 have been studied in DSRCT. Modak et al [150] has described 70% expression of G (D2) and 96% expression for 8H9 in 46 cases of DSRCT and both GD2 and the 58 kd antigen were localized to tumor cell membrane and stroma.GD2 is recognized by the monoclonal antibody 3F8, and a novel tumor antigen recognized by the mono clonal antibody 8H9 as two possible targets for immunotherapy of this tumor. Rachfal et al [151] showed in his study that connective tissue growth factor (CCN2) is expressed both by the tumor cells and supporting stromal fibroblasts and vascular endothelial cells and suggested that CCN2 is involved in autocrine and paracrine pathways of action. He further suggested that CCN2 expression is associated with the EWS-WT1 fusion, probably the inhibitory control of CCN2 gene expression by WT1 may be overcome by the pathological fusion of EWS to WT1, leading to localized CCN2 expression and the concomitant formation of desmoplastic stroma. Therefore CCN proteins may be useful targets for developing novel therapeutic approaches for treating DSRCT. Li et al [152] have demonstrated that ENT4 (equilibrative nucleoside transporter 4) is transcriptionally activated by both isoforms of EWS/WT1 and is highly expressed in DSRCT. It may represent an attractive pathway for targeting chemotherapeutic drugs.

# Chapter XII

# Prognosis

The prognosis of DSRCT is abysmal and despite multiple treatment strategies including several chemotherapy regimens, aggresive debulking surgery, abdominopelvic radiation, high-dose chemotherapy with autologous stem cell transplant followed by myeloablative therapy and stem cell rescue, there is no marked improvement in overall survival rate.

The average survival rate is 1.5-2.5 years and 15% overall survival at 5 years [138]. The results of combination of optimal cytoreductive surgey followed by multiagent chemotherapy resulted in a 3-year survival rate of 58% compared to inoperable patients [138]. Other authors found a median survival of 34 months compared to 14 months for operable and inoperable tumors, respectively [41].The longest survivor after the diagnosis of DSRCT was reported by Gil et al to be 101 months [20].

In most early reports, despite of aggressive surgical treatment and a complete response to chemotherapy most of the patients developed clinical relapse and there were no long term survivors. These patients die at a median of 17-25.5 months after the initial diagnosis. Ordonez et al [10] reported that 16 of 22 patients died of the disease within 8-50 months after initial therapy. Another study by Ordonez et al of 35 patients with follow-up information found that 25 died of widespread metastases and the remaining were alive with disease at a mean duration of 25.2 months. The median survival is less than 30 months in different studies with only 44% and 15% of patients alive at

3 and 5 years respectively after diagnosis [10,136,138]. A recent study in 18 Chinese patients with DSRCT showed the 1-year, 3-year, and 5-year survival rates to be 52.36%, 27.92%, and 27.92%, respectively [156].

Patients with hepatic parenchymal metastases have a dismal prognosis, with median survival of 18 months [136]. The cases reported by Alaggio et al [75] with morphological variation of DSRCT showed the longest survival of 13 years. Maximal multidisciplinary therapeutic approach has resulted in gratifying long-term survival to some extent but still DSRCT remains a devastating disease.

# Conclusion

In conclusion DSRCT has typical histological appearance and immunohistochemical profile. Additional ancillary techniques such as electron microscopy and cytogenetic studies would help to establish the correct diagnosis. Surgical excision is usually recommended for non-metastatic disease with combination chemo-radiotherapy as an adjunct. These tumors are highly chemosensitive therefore adjuvant chemotherapy is offered to all patients regardless of undergoing optimal or sub-optimal tumor resection.

Recent literature suggests that multidisciplinary treatment including high-dose chemotherapy, aggressive debulking surgery, radiation and myelo-ablative chemotherapy with stem cell rescue might be the proper approach to this rare malignancy and may improve progression-free survival.

# References

[1]    Gerald WL, Rosai J. Case 2: desmoplastic small cell tumor with divergent differentiation. *Pediatr Pathol* 1989; 9:177–183.

[2]    Gerald WL, Miller HK, Battifora H, Miettinen M, Silva EG, Rosai J. Intra-abdominal desmoplastic small round-cell tumor. Report of 19 cases of a distinctive type of high-grade polyphenotypic malignancy affecting young individuals. *Am J Surg Pathol* 1991; 15:499-513.

[3]    Sesterhenn I, Davis CJ, Mostofi FK. Undifferentiated malignant epithelial tumors involving serosal surfaces of scrotum and abdomen in young males. *J Urol* 1987; 137:214.

[4]    Gonzalez-Crussi F, Crawford SE, Sun CC. Intraabdominal desmoplastic small-cell tumors with divergent differentiation: observations on three cases of childhood. *Am J Surg Pathol.* 1990; 14:633–42.

[5]    Ordonez NG, Zirkin R, Bloom Re. Malignant small-cell epithelial tumor of the peritoneum co-expressing mesenchymal-type intermediate filaments. *Am J Surg Pathol* 1989; 13:413-21.

[6]    Wills EJ. Peritoneal desmoplastic small round cell tumors with divergent differentiation: A review. *Ultrastruc Pathol* 1993; 17:295-306.

[7]    Yaqoob N, Hasan SH. Desmoplastic small round cell tumour. *J Coll Physicians Surg Pak* 2006; 16:614-6.

[8]   Smith ME, Pelletier JP, Daniels R. A large abdominal mass in an otherwise healthy 31-year-old man. Intra- abdominal desmoplastic small round cell tumor. *Arch Pathol Lab Med* 2000; 124:1839-1840.

[9]   Lee SY, Hsiao CH. Desmoplastic small round cell tumor: A clinicopathologic, immunohistochemical and molecular study of four patients. *J Formos Med Assoc* 2007; 106:854-860.

[10]  Ordonez NG. Desmoplastic small round cell tumor-I: a histopathologic study of 39 cases with emphasis on unusual histologic patterns. *Am J Surg Pathol* 1998; 22:1303-1313.

[11]  Ordonez NG: Application of mesothelin immunostaining in tumor diagnosis. *Am J Surg Pathol* 2003;27:1418-28.

[12]  Choi JK, van Hoeven K, Brooks JJ, Gupta PK. Desmoplastic small round cell tumor presenting in pleural fluid and accompanied by Desmin-positive mesothelial cells. *Acta Cytol* 1995;39:377-378.

[13]  Mayall FG, Jasani B, Gibbs AR: Immunohistochemical positivity for neuron-specific enolase and Leu-7 in malignat mesotheliomas. *J Pathol* 1991;165:325-328.

[14]  Chang F. Desmoplastic small round cell tumors. Cytologic, histologic and immunohistochemical features. *Arch Pathol Lab Med.* 2006; 130:728-732.

[15]  Bland AE, Shah AA, Piscitelli JT, Bentley RC, Secord AA. Desmoplastic small round cell tumor masquerading as advanced ovarian cancer. *Int J Gynecol Cancer* 2008; 18:847-50.

[16]  Murphy AJ, Bishop K, Pereira C, MacNeill SC, Ho M, Zielenska M, Thorner PS. A new molecular variant of desmoplastic small round cell tumor: significance if WT1 immunostaining in this entity. *Human pathol* 2008; 39:1763-1770.

[17]  Mead M, Jones MA, Decain M, Tarraza HM. Intra-abdominal desmoplastic small round-cell tumor in a postmenopausal female. Report of a case and review of the literature. *Eur J Gynaecol Oncol.* 1994;15:267-71.

[18]  Fukunaga M, Endo Y, Takaki K, Ishikawa E, Ushigome S. Post menopausal intra abdominal desmoplastic small cell tumor. *Pathol Int.* 1996;46:281-5.

[19] Reich O, Justus J, Tamussino KF. Intra-abdominal desmoplastic small round cell tumor in a 68-year-old female. *Eur J Gynaecol Oncol* 2000; 21:126-7.

[20] Gill A, Gomez Portilla A, Brun EA, Sugarbaker PH. Clinical Perspective on desmoplastic small round-cell tumor. *Oncology* 2004; 67:231-42.

[21] Takahira K, Ohi S, Fujii N, Matsuura Y, Sano M, Hanai H, Kaneko E. Intra-abdominal desmoplastic small round cell tumor (IDSRT). *J Gastroenterol* 2000; 35: 712-716.

[22] Shintaku M, Baba Y, Fujiwara T. Intra-abdominal desmoplastic small cell tumor with Peutz-Jeghers syndrome. *Virchows Arch* 1994,425:211-215.

[23] Furman J, Murphy WM, Wajsman Z, Berry AD 3rd. Urogenital involvement by desmoplastic small round cell tumor. *J Urol* 1997;158:1506-09.

[24] Murosaki N, Matsumiya K, Kokado Y, Yoshioka T, Yasunaga Y, Aozasa K, Okuyama A. Retrovesical desmoplastic small round cell tumor in a patient with urinary frequency. *Int J Urol* 2001;8:245-8.

[25] Chang CC, Hsu JT, Tseng JH, Hwang TL, Chen HM, Jan YY. Combined resection and multi-agent adjuvant chemotherapy for desmoplastic small round cell tumor arising in the abdominal cavity: Report of a case. *World J Gastroenterol* 2006; 12:800-803.

[26] Tison V, Cerasoli S, Morigi F, Ladanyi M, Gerald WL, Rosai J. Intracranial desmoplastic small-cell tumor. *Am J Surg Pathol* 1996; 20:112-7.

[27] Neder L, Scheithauer BW, Turel KE, Arnesen MA, Ketterling RP, Jin L, Moynihan TJ, Giannini C, Meyer FB. Desmoplastic small round cell tumor of the central nervous system: report of two cases and review of literature. *Virchows Arch.* 2009;454(4):431-9.

[28] Bouchireb K, Auger N, Bhangoo R, Di Rocco F, Brousse N, Delattre O, Varlet P, Grill J. Intracerebral small round cell tumor: an unusual case with EWS-WT1 translocation. *Pediatr Blood Cancer* 2008;51(4):545-8.

[29] Wolf AN, Ladanyi M, Paull G, Blaugrund JE, Westra W. The expanding clinical spectrum of desmoplastic small round cell tumor: a report of

two cases with molecular confirmation. *Human Pathol* 1999;30(4):430-5.

[30]  Finke NM, Lae ME, Lloyd RV, Gehani SK, Nascimento AG. Sinonasal desmoplastic small round cell tumor: a case report. *Am J Surg Pathol.* 2002; 26:799-803.

[31]  Santos Gorjon P, Gomez Gonzalez JL, Batuecas Caletrio A, Flores Corral MT, Sanchez Gonzalez F. Small round cell desmoplastic tumour. Atypical morphology in the sub-maxillary gland. *Acta Otorrinolaringol* 2009;60(2):141-3.

[32]  Su MC, Jeng YM, Chu YC. Desmoplastic small round cell tumor of the kidney. *Am J Surg Pathol* 2004; 28:1379-1383.

[33]  Wang LL, Perlman EJ, Vujanic GM, Zuppan C, Brundler MA, Cheung CRH, Calicchio ML, Dubois S, Cendron M, Murata-collins JL, Wenger GD, Strzelecki D, Barr FG, Collins T, Perez-Atayde AR, Kozakewich H. Desmoplastic Small Round Cell Tumor of the Kidney in childhood. *Am J Surg Pathol* 2007; 31:576-584.

[34]  Collardeau-Frachon S, Ranchere-Vince D, Delattre O, Hoarau S, Thiesse P, Dubois R, Bergeron C, Dijoud F, Bouvier R. Primary Desmoplastic Small Round Cell Tumor of the Kidney: A Case Report in a 14-Year-Old Girl with Molecular Conformation. *Pediatr Dev Pathol* 2007; 10:320-324.

[35]  Egloff AM, Lee EY, Dillon JE, Callahan MJ. Desmoplastic small round cell tumor of the kidney in a pediatric patient: sonographic and multiphase CT findings. *Am J Roentgenol* 2005; 185:1347-1349.

[36]  Eaton SH, Cendron MA. Primary desmoplastic small round cell tumor of the kidney in a 7-year-old girl. *J Pediatr Urol.* 2006; 2:52-4.

[37]  Lee SB, Kolquist KA, Nichols K, Englert C, Maheswaran S, Ladanyi M, Gerald WL, Haber DA. The EWS-WT1 translocation product induces PDGFA in desmoplastic small round –cell tumor. *Nat Genet* 1997; 17:309-13.

[38]  Zhang PJ, Goldblum JR, Pawel BR, Pasha TL, Fisher C, Barr FG. PDGF-A, PDGF-R Beta, TGF- Beta3 and bone morphogenic protein-4 in desmoplastic small round cell tumors with EWS-WT1 gene fusion

product and their role in stromal desmoplasia: an immunohistochemical study. *Mod Pathol.* 2005; 18:382-387.

[39] Murphy A, Stallings RL, Howard J, O'Sullivan M, Hayes R, Breatnach F, McDermott MB. Primary desmoplastic small round cell tumor of bone: report of a case with cytogenetic confirmation. *Cancer Genet Cytogenet.* 2005; 156:167-171.

[40] Adsay V, Cheng J, Athanasian E, Gerald W, Rosai J. Primary desmoplastic small cell tumor of soft tissues and bone of the hand. Am J Surg Pathol. 1999; 23: 1408–1413. Tumor: report of a case. *Am J Surg Pathol.* 1996; 20:112–117.

[41] Biswas G, Laskar S, Banavali SD, Gujral S, Kurkure PA, Muckaden M, Parikh PM, Nair CN. Desmoplastic small round cell tumor: extra abdominal and abdominal presentations and the results of treatment. *Indian J Cancer* 2005; 42: 78-84.

[42] Yoshida A, Edgar MA, Garcia J, Meyers PA, Morris CD, Panicek DM. Primary desmoplastic small round cell tumor of the femur. *Skeletol Radiol* 2008;37(9):857-62.

[43] Zhao-ming W, Wen-bo X, Shu-sen Z. Desmoplastic small round cell tumor of the lung: case report. *Chinese Medical Journal* 2007; 120:2327-2328.

[44] Parkash V, Gerald WL, Parma A, Miettinen M, Rosai J. Desmoplastic small round cell tumor of the pleura. *Am J Surg Pathol* 1995;19:659-65.

[45] Syed S, Haque AK, Hawkins HK, Sorensen PH, Cowan DF. Desmoplastic small round cell tumor of the lung. *Arch Pathol Lab Med* 2002;126:1226-8.

[46] Sapi Z, Szentirmay Z, Orosz Z. Desmoplastic small round cell tumor of the pleura:a case report with further cytogenetic and ultrastructural evidence of 'mesothelioblastemic' origin. *Eurp J Surg Oncol* 1999; 25: 633-634.

[47] Ostoros G, Orosz Z, Kovacs G, Soltesz I. Desmoplastic small round cell tumor of the pleura: a case report with unusual follow-up. *Lung Cancer* 2002; 36: 333-6.

[48] Neuzillet C, Hammel P, Couvelard A, Msika S, Felce-Dachez M, Laé M, Lévy P, Ruszniewski P. Desmoplastic small round cell tumor of the

pancreas with breast metastasis. *Gastroenterol Clin Biol.* 2009;33:217-24.

[49] Bismar TA, Basturk O, Gerald WL, Schwarz K, Adsay NV. Desmoplastic Small cell tumor in the pancreas. *Am J Surg Pathol.* 2004; 28:808-12.

[50] Backer A, Mount SL, Zarka MA, Trask CE, Allen EF, Gerald WL, Sanders DA, Weaver DL. Desmoplastic small round cell tumour of unknown primary origin with lymph node and lung metastases: histological, cytological, ultrastructural, cytogenetic and molecular findings. *Virchows Arch* 1998;432:135-141.

[51] Kinra P, Pujahari AK. Desmoplastic small round cell tumor-abdomen. *Indian J Pathol Microbiol.* 2008; 51:449-50.

[52] Roganovich J, Bisogno G, Cecchetto G, D'Amore ES, Carli M. Paratesticular desmoplastic small round cell tumor: case report and review of the literature. *J Surg Oncol.*1999; 71:269-72.

[53] Garcia-Gonzalez J, Villanueva C, Fernandez-Acenero MJ, Paniagua P. Paratesticular desmoplastic small round cell tumor: case report. *Urol Oncol* 2005; 23:132-4.

[54] Bisogno G, Roganovich J, Sotti G, Ninfo V, di Montezemolo LC, Donfrancesco A, Mascarin M, Carli M. Desmoplastic small round cell tumour in children and adolescents. *Med Pediatr Oncol.* 2000;34 (5):338-42.

[55] Kawano N, Inayama Y, Nagashima Y, Miyagi Y, Uemura H, Saitoh K, Kubota Y, Hosaka M, Tanaka Y, Nakatami Y. Desmopalstic small round cell tumor of the paratesticular region: report of an adult case with demonstration of EWS and WT1 gene fusion using paraffin embedded tissue. *Mod Pathol* 1999; 12:729-734.

[56] Cummings OW, Ulbright TM, Young RH, Dei Tos AP, Fetcher CD, Hull MT. Desmoplastic small round cell tumors of the paratesticular region: a report of six cases. *Am J Surg Pathol* 1997; 21:219-25.

[57] Church DN, Bailey J, Hughes J, Williams CJ. Desmoplastic small round cell tumor: obstetric and gynecological presentations. *J Gynecol oncol.* 2006; 102: 583-6.

[58] Khalbuss WE, Bui M, Loya A. A 19-year-old woman with a cervicovaginal mass and elevated Serum CA 125. Desmoplastic small round cell tumor. *Arch Pathol Lab Med.* 2006; 130:59-61.

[59] Fang X, Rodabaugh K, Pnetrante R, Wong M, Wagner T, Sait S, Mhawech-Fauceglia P. Desmoplastic small round cell tumor (DSRCT) with ovarian involvement in 2 young women. *Appl Immunohistochem Mol Morphol* 2008; 16:94-9.

[60] Young RH, Eichhorn JH, Dickersin GR, Scully RE. Ovarian involvement by the intra abdominal desmoplastic small round cell tumor with divergent differentiation: A report of three cases. *Human Pathol.* 1992; 23: 454-64.

[61] Zaloudek C, Miller TR, Stern JL. Desmoplastic small cell tumor of the ovary; a unique polyphenotypic tumor with an unfavorable prognosis. *Int J Gynec Pathol.* 1995;14:260–5.

[62] Slomovitz BM, Girotra M, Aledo A, Saqi A, Soslow RA, Spigland NA, Caputo TA. Desmoplastic small round cell tumor with primary ovarian involvement: case report and review. *Gynec Oncol.* 2000; 79:124–8.

[63] Elhajj M, Mazurka J, Daya D. Desmplastic small round cell tumor presenting in the ovaries: report of a case and review of the literature. *Int J Gynecol. Cancer* 2002;12:760-3.

[64] Zeeshan-ud-din, Yaqoob N, Pishori T, Rafique AZ, Kamran A.Intra-abdominal desmoplastic small round cell tumor. *J Pak Med Assoc* 2006; 56:608-10.

[65] Parker LP, Duong JL, Wharton JT, Malpica A, Silva EG, Deavers MT. Desmoplastic small round cell tumor: report of a case presenting as a primary ovarian neoplasm. *Eur J Gynaecol Oncol* 2002; 23:199-202.

[66] Fizazi K, Farhat F, Theodore C, Rixe O, Le cesne A, Comoy E, Le Chevalier T. CA 125 and neuron specific enolase (NSE) as tumor markers for intra-abdominal desmoplastic small round cell tumors. *Br Jr cancer* 1997; 75(1):76-8.

[67] Yang SF, Wang SL, Chai CY, Su YC, Fu OY, Chen CY. Intra-abdominal desmoplastic small round cell tumor with elevated serum CA 125: a case report. *Kaohsiung J Med Sci* 2003; 19(10): 531- 6.

[68]  Ordonez NG, Sahin AA. CA 125 production in desmoplastic small round cell tumor: report of a case with elevated serum levels and prominent signet ring morphology. *Human Pathol* 1998; 29: 294-9.

[69]  Yoshizawa J, Maie M, Eto T, Higashimoto Y, Saito T, Horie H, Urano F. A case of intra-abdominal desmoplastic small round cell tumor with elevated serum CA 125. *Pediatr Surg Int.* 2002; 18: 238-40.

[70]  Motoyama T, Maejima T, Aizawa K, Fukuda T, Watanabe H. Biphasic intra abdominal desmoplastic small cell tumor in a patient with proximal spinal muscular atrophy. *Pathol Int.* 1996; 46:54-9.

[71]  Ordonez NG, El-Naggar AK, Ro JY, Silva EG, Mackay B. Intra-abdominal desmoplastic small cell tumor: a light microscopic, immunocytochemical, ultrastructural, and flow cytometric study. *Hum Pathol* 1994; 24:850-65.

[72]  Pasquinelli G, Montanaro L, Martinelli GN. Desmoplastic small round-cell tumor: a case report on the large cell variant with immunohistochemical, ultrastructural and molecular genetic analysis. *Ultrastruct Pathol* 2000, 24:333-7.

[73]  Dorsey BV, Benjamin LE, Rauscher F 3rd, Klencke B, Venook AP, Warren RS, Weidner N. Intra-abdominal desmoplastic small round-cell tumor: expansion of the pathologic profile. *Mod Pathol.* 1996; 9(6):703-9.

[74]  Zhang J, Dalton J, Fuller C. Epithelial marker- negative desmoplastic small round cell tumor with atypical morphology. *Arch Pathol Lab Med* 2007; 131:646-649.

[75]  Alaggio R, Rosolen A, Sartori F, Leszl A, d'Amore ESG, Bisogno G, Carli M, Cecchetto G, Coffin CM, Ninfo V. Spindle cell tumor with EWS-WT1 transcript and a favorable clinical course: A variant of DSCT, a variant of leiomyosarcoma, or a new entity? Report of 2 pediatric cases. *Am J Surg Pathol* 2007; 31:454- 459.

[76]  Gerald WL, Ladanyi M, de Alava E, Cuatrecasas M, Kushner BH, La Quaglia MP, Rosai J. Clinical, pathologic, and molecular spectrum of tumors associated with t(11;22)(p13;q12): desmoplastic small round cell tumor and its variants. *J Clin Oncol* 1998; 16:3028–3036.

[77] Ordonez NG. Desmoplastic small round cell tumor II: An ultrastructural and Immunohistochemical study with emphasis on new immunohistochemical markers. *Am J Surg Pathol* 1998; 22:1314-1327

[78] Lomovec J. Intra-abdominal desmoplastic small round cell tumour with expression of muscle specific actin. *Histopathology* 1994;24:577-9.

[79] Smithey B, Pappo As, Hill DA. C-Kit expression in pediatric solid tumors. A comparative Immunohistochemical study. *Am J Surg Pathol* 2002; 26(4): 486–92.

[80] Lae ME, Roche PC, Jin L, Lloyd RV, Nascimento AG. Desmoplastic small round cell tumor: a clinicopathologic, immunohistochemical and molecular study of 32 tumors. *Am J Surg Pathol* 2002; 26:823– 835.

[81] Trupiano JK, Machen SK, Barr FG, Goldblum JR. Cytokeratin-negative desmoplastic small round cell tumor: a report of two cases emphasizing the utility of reverse transcriptase-polymerase chain reaction. *Mod Pathol* 1999; 12: 849-53.

[82] Nishio J, Iwasaki H, Ishiguro M, fukuda T, Chuman H, Kaneko Y, Kikuchi M. Intra-abdominal small round cell tumour with EWS-WT1 fusion transcript in an elderly patient. *Histopathology* 2003; 42:404-12.

[83] Barnoud R, Sabourin JC, Pasquier D, Ranchere D, Bailly C, Lacombe MJT, Pasquier B. Immunohistochemical expression of WT1 by desmoplastic small round cell tumor. *Am J Surg Pathol* 2000; 24:830– 36.

[84] Hill DA, Pfeifer JD, Marley EF, Dehner LP, Humphrey PA, Zhu X, Swanson PE. WT1 staining reliably differentiates desmoplastic small round cell tumor from Ewings sarcoma/primitive neuroectodermal tumor. An immunohistochemical and molecular diagnostic study. *Am J Clin Pathol* 2000; 114(3):345-53.

[85] Zhang PJ, Goldblum JR, Pawel BR, Fisher C, Pasha TL, Barr FG. Immunophenotype of desmoplastic small round cell tumors as detected in cases with EWS-WT1 gene fusion product. *Mod Pathol* 2003; 16:229–35.

[86] Froberg K, Brown RE, Gaylord H, Manivel C. Intra-abdominal desmoplastic small round cell tumor: immunohistochemical evidence

for up-regulation of autocrine and paracrine growth factors. *Ann Clin Lab Sci* 1999; 29:78-85.

[87] Setrakian S, Gupta PK, Heald J, Brooks JJ. Intraabdominal desmoplastic small round cell tumor: report of a case diagnosed by fine-needle aspiration cytology. *Acta Cytol.* 1992; 36: 373-6.

[88] Caraway NP, Fanning CV, Amato RJ, Ordonez NG, Katz RL. Fine-needle aspiration of intra-abdominal desmoplastic small cell tumor. *Diagn Cytopathol* 1993;9:465-70.

[89] El-Kattan I, Redline RW, el-Naggar AK, Grimes MC, Abdul-Karim FW. Cytologic features of intraabdominal desmoplastic small round cell tumor. A case report. *Acta Cytol* 1995;39:514-20.

[90] Bian Y, Jordan AG, Rupp M, Cohn H, Mclaughlin CJ, Miettinen M. Effusion cytology of desmoplastic small round cell tumor of the pleura. A case report. *Acta Cytol* 1993; 37:77-82.

[91] Drut R. Biphasic intrabdominal desmoplastic small round cell tumor: fine needle aspiration cytology findings. *Diagn Cytopathol* 1995;13:325-32.

[92] Granja NM, Begnami MD, Bortolan J, Filho AL, Schmitt FC. Desmoplastic small round cell tumor: cytological and immuno-cytochemical features. *Cytojournal* 2005, 182(1):6.

[93] Dave B, Shet T, Chinoy R. Desmoplastic round cell tumor of childhood: can cytology with immunocytochemistry serve as an alternative for tissue diagnosis? *Diagn Cytopathol* 2005; 32: 330-5.

[94] Akhtar M, Ali MA, Sabbah R, Bakry M , al-Dayel F. Small round cell tumor with divergent differentiation: cytologic, histologic, and ultrastructural findings. *Diagn Cytopathol.* 1994; 11:159-164.

[95] Presley AE, Kong AE, Kong CS, Rowe DM, Atkins KA. Cytology of desmoplastic small round cell tumor: comparison of pre- and post-chemotherapy fine-needle aspiration biopsies. *Cancer* 2007; 111:41-6.

[96] Crapanzano JP. Cardillo M. Lin O, Zakowski MF. Cytology of desmoplastic small round cell tumor. *Cancer.*2002; 96:21-31.

[97] Pang B, Leong CC, Salto-Tellez M, Petersson F. Desmoplastic small round cell tumor of major salivary glands: report of 1 case and a review

of the literature. *Appl Immunohistochem Mol Morphol.* 2011 Jan;19(1):70-5.

[98] Outwater E, Scheibler ML, Brooks JJ. Intraabdominal desmoplastic small cell tumor: CT and MR findings. *J Comput Assist Tomogr* 1992; 16:429-432.

[99] Kretschmar CS, Colbach C, Bhan I, Crombleholme TM. Desmoplastic small cell tumor: a report of three cases and a review of the literature. *J Pediatr Hematol Oncol* 1996; 18:293-8.

[100] Meyers MA. Dynamic radiology of the abdomen: normal and pathologic anatomy. New York, NY: Springer-Verlag, 2000.

[101] Pickhardt PJ, Fisher AJ, Balfe DM, Dehner LP, Huettner PC. Desmoplastic small round cell tumor of the abdomen: radiologic-histopathologic correlation. *Radiology* 1999;210:633–638.

[102] Bellah R, Suzuki-Bordalo L, Brecher E, Ginsberg JP, Maris J, Pawel BR. Desmoplastic small round cell tumor in the abdomen and pelvis: report of CT findings in 11 affected children and young adults. *AJR Am J Roentgenol* 2005;184:1910-4.

[103] Sabate JM, Torrubia S, Roson N, Matias-Guiu X, Gomez A. Intra-abdominal desmoplastic small round-cell tumor: a rare cause of peritoneal malignancy in young people. *Eur Radiol* 2000;10:817-9.

[104] Gorospe L, Gomez T, Gonzalez LM, Lopez A. Desmoplastic small round cell tumor of the pelvis: MRI findings with histopathologic correlation. *Eur Radiol* 2007;17:287-8.

[105] Tateishi U, Hasegawa T, Kusumoto M, Oyama T, Ishikawa H, Moriyama N. Desmoplastic small round cell tumor: imaging findings associated with clinicopathologic features. *J Comput Assist Tomogr* 2002;26:579-83.

[106] Pickhardt PJ. F-18 fluorodeoxyglucose Positron Emission Tomographic Imaging of the Desmoplastic Small Round Cell Tumor of the Abdomen. *Clin Nucl Med* 1999;24:693-94.

[107] Mayall FG, Gibbs AR. The histology and immunohistochemistry of small cell mesothelioma. *Histopathology* 1992;20:47–51.

[108] Einstein DM, Tagliabue JR, Desai RK. Abdominal desmoids: CT findings in 25 patients. *AJR* 1991; 157:275-279.

[109] Maillard JC, Menu Y, Scerrer A, et al. Intraperitoneal splenosis: diagnosis by ultrasound and computed tomography. *Gastrointest Radiol* 1989; 14:179-180.

[110] Ferreiros J, Leon NG, Mata MI, et al. Computer tomography in abdominal Castleman's disease. *J Comput Assist Tomogr* 1989; 13:433-436.

[111] Leder RA, Low VHS. Tuberculosis of the abdomen. *Radiol Clin North Am* 1995; 33:691-703.

[112] Chan Y, Cheng CSK, Ng P. Mesenteric actinomycosis. *Abdom Imaging* 1993; 18:286-287.

[113] Papadatos D, Taourel P, Bret PM. CT of leiomyomatosis peritonealis disseminata mimicking peritoneal carcinomatosis. *AJR* 1996; 167:475-476.

[114] McCluggage WG, Oliva E, Connolly LE, McBride HA, Young RH. An immunohistochemical analysis of ovarian small cell carcinoma of hypercalcemic type. *Int J Gynecol Pathol* 2004;23:330-336.

[115] Yachnis AT, Rorke LB, Biegel JA, Peirlongo G, Zimmerman RA, Sutton LN. Desmoplastic primitive neuroectodermal tumor with divergent differentiation. Broadening the spectrum of desmoplastic infantile neuroepithelial tumors. *Am J Surg Pathol* 1992;16:998-1006.

[116] Leuschner I, Newton WA, Schmidt Det al. Spindle cell variants of Embryonal rhabdomyosarcoma in the paratesticular region. *Am J Surg Pathol.* 1993; 17:221-230.

[117] Sawyer JR, Tryka AF, Lewis JM. A novel reciprocal chromosome translocation t(11;22)(p13;q12) in an intraabdominal desmoplastic small round-cell tumor. *Am J Surg Pathol.* 1992;16:411-6.

[118] Biegel JA, Conard K, Brooks JJ. Translocation (11;22) (p13;q12):primary change in intra-abdominal desmoplastic small round cell tumor. *Genes Chromosomes Cancer* 1993;7:119-21.

[119] Rodriguez E, Sreekantaiah C, Gerald W, Reuter VE, Motzer RJ, Chaganti RS. *A recurring translocation,* t(11;22)(p13;q11.2), characterizes intra-abdominal desmoplastic small round cell tumors. *Cancer Genet. Cytogenet.* 1993;69:17-21.

[120] de Alava E, Ladanyi M, Rosai J, Gerald WL. Detection of chimeric transcripts in desmoplastic small round cell tumor and related developmental tumors by reverse transcriptase polymerase chain reaction: a specific diagnostic assay. *Am J Pathol* 1995; 147:1584-91.

[121] Argatoff LH, O'Connell JX, Mathers JA, Gilks CB, Sorensen PHB. Detection of the EWS/WT1 gene fusion by reverse transcriptase polymerase chain reaction in the intra-abdominal desmoplastic small round cell tumor. *Am J Surg Pathol* 1996; 20:406-12.

[122] Antonesue CR, Gerald WL, Magid MS, Ladanyi M. Molecular variants of the EWS-WT1 gene fusion in desmoplastic small round cell tumor. *Diagn Mol Pathol* 1998; 7:24-8.

[123] Hamazaki M, Okita H, Hata J, Shimizu S, Kobayashi H, Aoki K, Nara T. Desmoplastic small cell tumor of soft tissue: molecular variant of EWS-WT1 chimeric fusion. *Pathol Int* 2006; 56:543-8.

[124] Ordi J, de Alava E, Torne A, Mellado B, Pardo Mindan J, Iglesias X, Cardesa A. Intrabdominal Desmoplastic small round cell tumor with EWS/ERG fusion transcript. *Am J Surg Pathol* 1998; 22(8):1026-32.

[125] Katz RL, Quezado M, Senderowicz AM, Villalba L, Laskin WB, Tsokos M. An intra-abdominal small round cell neoplasm with features of primitive neuroectodermal and desmoplastic round cell tumor and a EWS/FLI-1 fusion transcript. *Hum Pathol* 1997; 28: 502-9.

[126] Thorner P. Intra-abdominal polyphenotypic tumor. *Pediatr Pathol Lab Med.* 1996;16:161-9.

[127] Thorner P, Squire J, Chilton-MacNeil S,et al. Is the EWS/FL1 fusion transcript specific for Ewings sarcoma and peripheral primitive neuroectodermal tumor? A report of four cases showing this transcript in a wider range of tumor types. *Am J Surg Pathol* 1996:148:1125-38.

[128] Karnieli E, Werner H, Rauscher III FJ, Benjamin LE, Le Roith D. The IGF-I receptor gene promoter is a molecular target for the Ewing's Sarcoma-Wilms' tumor 1 fusion protein. *J Biol Chem* 1996; 271:19304-9.

[129] Werner H, Idelman G, Rubinstein M, Pattee P, Nagalla SR, Roberts CT Jr. A novel EWS-WT1 gene fusion product in desmoplastic small round

cell tumor is a potent transactivator of the insulin-like growth factor-I receptor (IGF-IR) gene. *Cancer Lett* 2007;247:84-90.

[130] Liu J, Nau MM, Yeh JC, Allegra CJ, Chu E, Wright JJ. Molecular heterogeneity and function of EWS-WT1 fusion transcripts in desmoplastic small round cell tumors. *Clin Cancer Res.* 2000;6:3522-9.

[131] Nishio J, Iwasaki H, Ishiguro M, Ohjimi Y, Fujita C, Yanai F, Nibu K, Mitsudome A, Kaneko Y, Kikuchi M. Establishment and characterization of a novel human desmoplastic small round cell tumor cell line, JN-DSRCT-1. *Lab Invest2002*; 82:1175-82.

[132] Ladanyi M, Gerald W. Fusion of the EWS and WT1 genes in the desmoplastic small round cell tumor. *Cancer Res* 1994;54:2837-40.

[133] Gerald W, Rosai J, Ladanyi M. Characterization of the genomic breakpoint and chimeric transcripts in the EWS-WT1 gene fusion of desmoplastic small round cell tumor. *Proc Natl Acad Sci* USA 1995;92:1028-32.

[134] Gerald WL, Haber DA. The EWS-WT1 gene fusion in desmoplastic small round cell tumor. *Semin Cancer Biol* 2005; 15:197-205.

[135] Livaditi E, Mavridis G, Soutis M, Papandreou E, Moschovi M, Papadakis V, Stefanaki K, Christopoulos-Geroulanos G. Diffuse intraabdominal desmoplastic small round cell tumour: a ten-year experience. *Eur J Pediatr Surg* 2006;16:423-7.

[136] La Quaglia MP, Brennan MF. The clinical approach to desmoplastic small round cell tumor. *Surg Oncol* 2000; 9:77-81.

[137] Hassan IS R, Donohue JH, Edmonson JH, Gunderson LL, Mrir CR, Arndt CA, Nascimento AG, Que FG. Intra-abdominal desmoplastic small round cell tumors: a diagnostic and therapeutic challenge. *Cancer* 2005; 104:1264-70.

[138] Lal DR, Su WT, Wolden SL, Loh KC, Modak S, La Quaglia MP. Results of multimodal treatment for desmoplastic small round cell tumors. *J Pediatr Surg* 2005; 40:251-5.

[139] Farhat F, Culine S, Lhomme C, Duvillard P, Soulie P, Michel G, Terrier-Lacombe MJ, Theodore C, Schreinerova M, Droz JP. Desmoplastic small round cell tumors: results of a four-drug chemotherapy regimen in five adult patients. *Cancer* 1996; 77:1363-6.

[140] Kushner BH, La Quaglia MP, Wollner N, Meyers PA, Lindsley KL, Gharimi F, Merchant TE, Boulad F, Cheung NK, Bonilla MA, Crouch G, Kelleher JF Jr, Steinherz PG, Gerald WL. Desmoplastic small round cell tumor: prolonged progression free survival with aggressive multimodality therapy. *J Clin Oncol* 1996; 14:1526-31.

[141] Kurre P, Felgenhauer JL, Miser JS, Patterson K, Hawkins DS. Successful dose-intensive treatment of desmoplastic small round cell tumor in three children. *J Pediatr hematol Oncol* 2000;22:446-50.

[142] Bertuzzi A, Castagna L, Quagliuolo V, Ginanni V, Compasso S, Magagnoli M, Balzarotti M, Nozza A, Siracusano L, Timofeeva I, Sarina B, Parra HS, Santoro A. Prospective study of high-dose chemotherapy and autologous peripheral stem cell transplantation in adult patients with advanced desmoplastic small round cell tumour. *Br Jr Cancer.* 2003;89:1159-61.

[143] Aguilera D, Hayes-Jordan A, Anderson P, Woo S, Pearson M, Green H. Outpatient and home chemotherapy with novel local control strategies in desmoplastic small round cell tumor. *Sarcoma* 2008;2008:261589.

[144] Goodman KA, Wolden SL, La Quaglia MP, Kushner BH. Whole abdomino-pelvic radiotherapy for desmoplastic small round cell tumor. *Int. J Radiat. Oncol. Biol. Phys.* 2002;54:170-176.

[145] Stuart-Buttle CE, Smart CJ, Pritchard S, Martin D, Welch IM. Desmoplastic small round cell tumor: A review of literature and treatment options. *Surg Oncol* 2008;17:107-12.

[146] Adamson PC, Blaney SM, Widemann BC, Kitchen B, Murphy RF, Hannah AL, Cropp GF, Patel M, Gillespie AF, Whitcomb PG, Balis FM. Pediatric phase I trial and pharmacokinetic study of the platelet-derived growth factor (PDGF) receptor pathway inhibitor SU101. *Cancer Chemother Pharmacol* 2004;53:482–8.

[147] Bond M, Bernstein ML, Pappo A, Schultz KR, Krailo M, Blaney SM, Adamson PC. A Phase 2 trial of Imatinib mesylate (IM) in children with refractory or relapsed solid tumors; a Children's Oncology Group Study. *Pediatr Blood Cancer* 2008;50:254-8.

[148] Mazuryk M, Paterson AH, Temple W, Arthur K, Crabtree T, Stewart DA. Benefit of aggressive multimodality therapy with autologous stem

cell support for intra-abdominal desmoplastic small round cell tumor. *Bone Marrow Transplant* 1998;21(9):961–3.

[149] Al-Balushi Z, Bulduc S, Mulleur C, Lallier M. Desmoplastic small round cell tumor in children: a new therapeutic approach. *J Pediatr Surg* 2009;44:949-52.

[150] Modak S, Kramer K, Gultekin SH, Guo HF, Cheung NK. Monoclonal antibody 8H9 targets a novel cell surface antigen expressed by a wide spectrum of human solid tumors. *Cancer Res* 2001;61(10): 4048–54.

[151] Rachfal AW, Luquette MH, Brigstock DR. Expression of connective tissue growth factor (CCN2) in desmoplastic small round cell tumor. *J Clin* Pathol 2004;57:422-5.

[152] Li H, Smolen GA, Beers LF, Xia L, Gerald W, Wang J, Harber DA, Lee SB. Adenosine transporter ENT4 is a direct target of EWS/WT1 translocation product and is highly expressed in desmoplastic small round cell tumor. *PLos One* 2008;3;6:e2353.

[153] Liping Cao, Jun Ni, Risheng Que, Zhengrong Wu, Zhenya Song. Desmoplastic small round cell tumor: a clinical, pathological, and immunohistochemical study of 18 Chinese cases. *Int J Surg Pathol* 2008;16(3):257-62.

[154] Kuhnen C, Schäfer KL, Franke K, Poremba C. *Cystic desmoplastic small round cell tumor: Tumor development from cystic-"mesothelioblastic" areas?* 2010 Jan 13. [Epub ahead of print]

[155] da Silva RC, Medeiros Filho P, Chioato L, Silva TR, Ribeiro SM, Bacchi CE. Desmoplastic small round cell tumor of the kidney mimicking Wilms tumor: a case report and review of the literature. *Appl Immunohistochem Mol Morphol* 2009;17:557-62.

[156] Engohan-Aloghe C, Aubain Sommerhausen Nde S, Noël JC. Ovarian involvement by desmoplastic small round cell tumor with leydig cell hyperplasia showing an unusual immunophenotype (cytokeratin negative, calretinin and inhibin positive) mimicking poorly differentiated sertoli leydig cell tumor. *Int J Gynecol Pathol* 2009; 28:579-83.

# Index

**D**

**E**